Why Do I Need Whole Food Supplements?

What everyone must know about the vitamins they are taking

by

Lorrie Medford, C.N.

LDN Publishing
P.O. Box 54007
Tulsa, Oklahoma 74155

WHY DO I NEED WHOLE FOOD SUPPLEMENTS?
What everyone must know about the vitamins they are taking
ISBN #978-0-9676419-3-5
Copyright © 2002 Lorrie Medford, C.N.
LDN Publishing
P. O. Box 54007
Tulsa, OK 74155

Library of Congress Cataloging-in-Publishing Data

Medford, Lorrie

> Why Do I Need Whole Food Supplements?
> Lorrie Medford, C.N.
> International Standard Book Number: 0-9676419-3-4
> 1. Nutrition 2. Health 3. Food Supplements I.Title

NOTE: This book is not intended to take the place of medical advice. Readers are advised to consult their doctor or other qualified healthcare professional regarding treatment of their medical conditions.

Printed in the United States of America

Fifth printing, 2010

(For ordering information, refer to the back pages of this book.)

The names of my clients have been changed. Any similarity to a real person is purely coincidental.

The doctor of the future will give no medicine but will interest his patients in the care of the human frame, in diet, and in the cause and prevention of disease.

Thomas Edison

Dedication

To the health professionals involved with whole-food supplements who understand how God made nutrients for our health, and care enough to give their patients the safest and most effective supplements.

To our clients who give us purpose in life. My sincere prayers for you for true health and fitness.

Contents

Foreword

For the first three years of being in the field of practicing nutrition and health, I felt diet and lifestyle change was all that was necessary for my patients to return to health. After three years it became apparent, for many of the reasons listed in this book, that my patients would need supplements to provide what the body needed to restore health. However, two more years passed before I prescribed one supplement. Why?

Because of my nutritional studies, I had learned that the supplements on the market were largely highly processed and of little value, if not actually harmful to the body, even with the word **natural** boldly printed on the label. In good conscience I could not recommend them. If my patients were going to put out money for health, then I wanted them to get their money's worth. As one researcher said, "Taking processed vitamins is like eating a banana peel and thinking you've just consumed a whole banana."

You can't afford **not** to read and use this book. Your health depends on it, never mind your pocketbook. Every year millions of dollars are spent on vitamin/mineral supplements, but in most cases the only people winning are the processed vitamin companies. If you haven't figured it out by now, you will as you read this book— the processed vitamin manufacturers are not interested in your health; they are interested in your pocket book.

After using whole-food supplements, the difference in my patient's progress was amazing. The best part about taking whole-food supplements, along with a healthy change in lifestyle, is that they balance the deficiencies. Then the patient is able to reduce how much they are taking (and spending) on supplements.

Lorrie Medford has done a masterful job with this book to not only help you understand the need for supplementation, but she also gives you the do's and don'ts when it comes to purchasing and using supplements. If you have wondered about the controversy over why you need supplements and what you need, this book will go far to help you understand.

Joel R. Robbins, D.C., M.D., N.D.
The Health and Wellness Center
Tulsa, Oklahoma

Every day I talk to patients who are confused, bewildered, and just plain angry about the amount of money they have spent on vitamins, minerals, "miracle cures," and everything else touted in those flashy newspapers waiting for us all at the grocery store check-out counter. You know the ones; you've picked them up and had a look. "Wow! Look at those before and after pictures! Sounds good; let's try one more time."

Advertising IS powerful and we ARE gullible. We are also sick and getting sicker. It is time for the simple truth about food and food supplements. It is time for healing and recovery from a lifetime of nutritional deficiencies that only whole, natural foods can provide.

Lorrie Medford's wonderful book will give YOU the information you need to make changes NOW. Lorrie gets right to the heart of the issue and explodes the myths that have been fostered on the American public by those who are, perhaps, motivated by less than the highest goals. If you are tired of being tired, if you are fed up with being overfed and undernourished, then Lorrie's straight-forward recommendations are exactly what you need. Read this book and give copies to all whose health is as important to you as your own. You and they will be glad you did!

Michael D. Dobbins, D. C.
Dobbins Affordable Chiropractic
Alameda, California

Acknowledgements

Many thanks to all of my clients who motivate me to continue to research, study and write. I pray that this book will answer the questions about supplements that you so frequently ask me. Special thanks to the clients who gave me their health testimonies to use in this book.

Special thanks also to Anne Spears, Carolyn Clark, Cathy Newcomer, Lori Oller, and Annette Ahalt, my wonderful assistants. You all have been involved in creating this book and I am grateful for your participation. I am most grateful to Lori, Cathy, and my twin sister, Jackie Johnson, for your outstanding editing and proofreading skills.

Many thanks to Tim Jurgensen for your excellent work on the cover.

I am grateful to all of the authors whom I have quoted, especially Dr. Royal Lee for his great passion and commitment to keeping people healthy. His heart was to give the public what they needed the most: whole-food nutrition. Not only was he a human rights advocate, he was also one of the most incredible nutritional geniuses of the century. Yet, he unfortunately had to spend countless hours fighting the FDA, trying to get the right to advertise his natural products while at the same time, large commercial industries promoted their devitalized foods. Yet Dr. Lee was the one who was persecuted. What a shame he had to fight for the right to heal people naturally when it should always be one of our greatest freedoms.

Many thanks to author Judith DeCava for her in-depth research on vitamins and how they are manufactured.

Thank you to Dr. Joel Robbins for being generous with your time and allowing me to interview you about the differences between whole-food supplements and synthetic vitamins, the fallacy of high-potency vitamins, and the labeling ploys used by some manufacturers. Thank you, too, for your foreword, helpful comments and for your gracious support and encouragement throughout the years.

Thank you to Dr. Michael Dobbins for reviewing my manuscript, writing your foreword, and offering valuable feedback. Thanks so much, too, for your faithfulness to teach seminars for healthcare professionals around the country nearly every weekend. All of our clients benefit from your research. And thanks for making it fun with your incredible sense of humor. (Wish you would sing for us sometime!)

Thanks too, to several people who reviewed my book and for all of your great comments and suggestions:

Charles DuBois—thanks for your incredible support and for keeping us healthy with the best supplements on the market.

Dr. Ray Bisesi for your help in reviewing articles from Dr. Royal Lee's archives.

And many thanks to several people who took time out of their busy schedules to review my book: Dr. Don Warren, Dr. Jim Rhodes, Dr. Andre Kulisz, Dr. Clyde Jensen, Dr. Bruce West, Tim Bahan, Hugh St. Onge, Glenn Kikel, and Vicki O'Brien. Special thanks to Walter Scott for your continual encouragement and support.

And finally, I thank God, without Whom I would not know, nor have, anything. Without You I would not know how to pursue life or my purpose for living.

About the Author

Author and motivational speaker, Lorrie Medford has a B.A. in Communications and is a licensed Certified Nutritionist from The American Health Science University. She also holds certification as a personal trainer from ISSA (International Sports Science Association). She serves on the Board of Directors for the Society of Certified Nutritionists, and is a member of the Oklahoma Speaker's Association. Lorrie also serves on the Advisory Board for Standard Process, Inc.

In addition to writing this book, she has also written *Why Can't I Stay Motivated?*, *Why Can't I Lose Weight?*, *Why Can't I Lose Weight Cookbook*, *Why Do I Feel So Lousy?*, *Why Am I So Grumpy, Dopey and Sleepy?*, *Why Am I So Wacky,* and *Why Eat Like Jesus Ate?*

A health researcher and journalist, Lorrie has studied nutrition, whole-foods cooking, herbs, health, fitness, and motivation for more than 20 years. Lorrie taught her weight-loss class at a local junior college and through her own business for more than 10 years, and has taught natural foods cooking classes in Spokane, Washington and Tulsa, Oklahoma for more than 5 years.

She shares her knowledge in her seminars, and through her thriving nutritional consultation practice, *Life Design Nutrition* in Tulsa, Oklahoma.

Lorrie has a rich history of community involvement teaching nutrition and is a sought-after speaker for civic groups, churches, hospitals, and wellness organizations.

She is uniquely qualified to write about health and fitness. Lorrie knows what it's like to be a *cranky calorie counter* obsessed with foods, dieting, and striving to be thin. After struggling with her weight for many years, Lorrie lost more than 35 pounds and has kept it off for more than nineteen years.

Are You Confused?

Being a health consumer is harder than ever. One day you might read an article in the magazine section of the Sunday paper that says how effective vitamin A is for preventing cancer. The next day, you hear on the late night news that taking vitamin A is toxic and can even cause cancer! Totally confused, you wonder who to believe. And that's how you start your collection.

We all have them. I did and most of my clients do, too. I am talking about all of those vitamin pill bottles that you have in the kitchen cupboard—stuff you've bought over the years, but probably stopped taking. People have a hard time throwing them away because they spent money on them. Who knows? Perhaps they could use them in an art project or something! (That was me—but more about that in my forthcoming book, *Why Can't I Throw Things Away?*)

Buying vitamins has become incredibly crazy. It's not like in the good old days, when there was only one type of multiple, vitamin or mineral. Today, there are fifteen different kinds of each. Once you figure out what you want and need, after reading every label for the past three hours, (where are the sales people when you need them?) then you find a supplement that combines several of them, but not all of them. Now you have to start all over, wondering "What's the difference between all these supplements anyway?" No wonder people are confused!

If You Feel Confused, You Are Not Alone

Most of my clients come in with a basket or two of vitamins that they have been collecting. Since they are coming to me, I always ask them if their supplements made them feel better. They usually say, "No," adding how frustrating it is to spend so much money on vitamins without any results. (This puts no pressure on me, of course!)

When I started my practice, I ordered vitamins I thought were good. But when my clients returned for their follow-ups, they didn't seem to be getting better. My first six months in practice, I sent dozens of unopened bottles back to various vitamin companies. I kept looking for whole-food supplements and talking to other nutritionists along the way. Some told me, "Oh, it doesn't matter; just buy so-and-so and you'll get a greater profit." But it did matter. I wasn't looking for the highest profit—I was looking for the best results.

I spoke to a fellow nutritionist at a seminar in California who told me, "I use some vitamins that work. I know they work because I saw the results with blood tests." Her results got my attention. I began using whole-food supplements and was amazed with the results. Now I'm not throwing away supplements anymore; but I have been known to give them away! Now it's unusual if we don't see our clients progressively improving their health.

Three Important Questions

Like many health professionals around the country, I have a wide variety of clients, both male and female ranging from housewives to business executives. Or, they could be students, athletes, or small children. No matter why they come to see me, they frequently ask me the same questions:

1. Why do I need vitamins and how long do I need them?

2. I already have a vitamin from a reputable company; why should I try what you recommend?

And I especially like the third question:

3. Can I take them with my donut and coffee in the mornings?

Where Do You Need Help?

Most people don't have the time to thoroughly investigate vitamins or get the right information to make wise selections. (But they do, apparently, have time to watch infomercials at 2:00 in the morning, which have become the source for all nutritional miracle breakthroughs!)

I've seen thousands of clients in my practice. From working with so many people, I've learned what supplements can and cannot do. In this book, I'll give you important reasons why we not only need supplements, but why they need to be whole-food supplements. Here's a review of the three parts of this book and their chapters.

Part One tells you about the status of American health.
1. Is America healthy? Are you?
2. Who decided what we should eat?
3. Who decided how many vitamins we need?

Part Two tells you why we need supplements.
4. Five reasons why we need to supplement our diet.
5. How food processing has damaged our health.
6. Why good soil is so vital for our health.

Part Three tells you how to buy supplements.
7. The difference between various supplements.
8. How synthetic vitamins can hurt you.
9. Potency: How much is enough?
10. What supplements do you really need?

Okay, let's move on to chapter one. Are we really a healthy nation?

PART ONE

Are We Really Healthy?

Can You Pass This Test?

As I was counseling John, a client of mine, I thought, "This guy is really healthy." His paperwork showed no real problems or health symptoms. I finally asked him, "Just why are you here?" He replied, "My wife made me come." Knowing that many men, of their own accord, won't even go to a doctor (unless their leg was shot and it's beginning to fall off their body) much less a nutritionist, I smiled at his wife's wisdom and said, "Fine—even though you are pretty healthy, let's see if there's anything I can do for you."

Then I asked a series of questions checking his vitamin status, and then his health, including frequency of headaches, sinus infections, joint problems, digestive problems, low energy level, and lack of sleep all to which he replied "Yes—he was healthy, except for all of those problems!" We helped him so much over the next few months, he even told his co-workers about us.

What About You?

Are you "healthy," except for those chronic infections, or earaches, allergies, toothaches, bladder infections, and so on? Yet each little ailment we experience is our body trying to tell us about some nutritional deficiency. How often do we settle for less than perfect health?

The World Health Organization has a great definition of health: "A state of complete physical, mental, and social well-being and not merely the absence of disease or infirmity." This definition has not been amended since 1948![1]

Your body tries to make new cells every day. Without proper nutrition it can't make healthy cells. So the next generation of cells is weaker. This is the beginning of disease.

You can witness the regenerative or healing power in your body any time you cut your finger. You don't have to "do" anything to heal it. Just clean your finger, and your body does the healing. The question always is, "Does your body have adequate nutrition to heal?"

We were designed to live long, healthy lives. If we're not healthy, somewhere along the way we have interfered with our healing process. We accept common symptoms listed previously as "normal" because everyone our age has them. But they are not normal—any more than it's normal for children and teens to get arthritis and heart disease. One hundred years ago this was unheard of. Why is it "normal" now? It's not normal; it's common now because children and teens are not getting the nutrition their grandparents did.

Let's Go Back in Time

In the beginning, most people died from being eaten by a wild animal, such as a dinosaur or some other unfortunate circumstance. But I understand other than that, they were pretty healthy!

Let's go back fifty years ago, when the big killer diseases were smallpox, diphtheria and tuberculosis. These illnesses were caused by infectious bacteria due to unsanitary living conditions and malnutrition. Once these conditions improved, health was restored. Next came chemically-preserved, processed foods which brought us to another state of malnutrition. There was no reported incidence of heart disease until the early 1900s and only 3% of Americans died from cancer.

What About Today?

Today, the top three killers include cancer, heart disease and diabetes. These diseases are not caused by bacteria, but nutritional deficiencies and chemical toxicity. The medical care costs for Americans with chronic diseases such as these totals more than $400 billion annually.

The National Center for Health Statistics gave the ten leading causes of death in the U.S. for the year 2000: Here are some of their findings.[2]

1. About 709,894 people died from heart disease. Heart disease is still the nation's number one cause of death.

2. About 551,833 people died from cancer.

According to Dr. Patrick Quillin in his revised edition of *Beating Cancer With Nutrition*, nearly half of our population can expect to develop cancer:

> Over 4 million Americans are currently being treated for cancer with another 4 million in remission, and possibly awaiting a recurrence of the cancer... Each year over 1.4 million more Americans are newly diagnosed with cancer. Forty-two percent of Americans living today can expect to develop cancer in his or her lifetime. **At least 40% of cancer patients will die from malnutrition, not the cancer itself.**[3]

The World Health Organization (WHO) estimates deaths from cancer will double over the next 20 years.[4]

3. About 68,662 people die from diabetes. In 2000, diabetes was the nation's sixth cause of death, associated with excessive calories and obesity. In addition, there are about eight million undiagnosed diabetics.

And today, obesity affects between 45-50 percent of the North American population; 13 percent of children in America are obese. My, how things have changed!

But there's so much more. In the United States, over 100 million people suffer from chronic pain. We gobble up billions of pain reliever pills to the tune of $30 billion a year.[5]

Unfortunately, most of this pain started out as some type of nutritional imbalance which could be handled with whole-food nutritional supplements, dietary changes and even whole-food herbal supplements—at half the cost of the pain relievers.

The Most Important Factor

Now we know that many of these deaths could have been prevented with proper nutrition and lifestyle! For the past twenty years, a tremendous amount of research has proved that malnutrition is a major contributor to disease and that proper nutrition can help **prevent** disease.

For example, nearly all fruits and vegetables are packed with antioxidants which defend our cells against attack by free radicals. Free radicals are the chemicals that damage and destroy cells, promoting aging and disease.

Certain vegetables and fruits can increase our immunity against heart disease, and help lower cholesterol. (If we could only get your family to squeeze them in between their French fries and burgers!) They can help reduce the incidence of breast, prostate and colon cancers. Broccoli, cabbage and cauliflower, for example, have phytochemical compounds that boost the production of anti-cancer enzymes within hours of being eaten. (Too bad they don't taste like pizza!)

Wisdom That Lasts

I framed Thomas Edison's famous quote which hangs in my office: *"The doctor of the future will give no medicine but will interest his patients in the care of the human frame, in diet, and in the cause and prevention of disease."* Solid research on nutrition and disease backs his age-old wisdom.

How Healthy Are You?

What about you? Do you jump out of bed every day, or does your spouse or other family member drag you out of bed? Do you need naps every day? Do you get colds often? Do you have pain anywhere? How safe are you from being one of these earlier mentioned statistics? What are you doing to prevent major diseases?

Let's take a quick look at **your** health. I've written a quick nutrition test for possible vitamin/mineral deficiencies. Score yourself this way.

No = 0 points Sometimes = 1 point Often = 2 points

Nutrition Test

1. Do you get infections like the flu, colds, and sore throats easily?
2. Do you have depression, irritability or anxiety? Do you experience great physical or emotional stress?
3. Do you have a high homocysteine level or heart disease? (Do you even know what homocysteine is?*)
4. Do you have pernicious anemia?
5. Do you bruise easily, have varicose veins, or bleeding gums?
6. Do you have problems with teeth, do you have soft nails or soft bones (rickets)?
7. Do you have fibrocystic breast disease?
8. Do you have trouble with blood clotting?
9. Do you have twitching muscles or leg cramps ?
10. Do you have hypoglycemia or sugar cravings?
11. Do you have high cholesterol (related to an imbalance of zinc)?
12. Do you have thyroid problems?
13. Do you crave chocolate?
14. Do you have arthritis, joint pain or clicking joints?
15. Do you have edema (swelling)?
16. Do you have prostate problems or low resistance to colds or flu?

Possible Vitamin/Mineral Deficiencies

Here are common vitamins or minerals that you could be deficient in if you answered yes to any of the questions above.

1. Vitamin A
2. B complex (includes all B vitamins)
3. Folic acid
4. Cobalamin or B12
5. Vitamin C
6. Vitamin D
7. Vitamin E
8. Vitamin K
9. Calcium
10. Chromium
11. Copper
12. Iodine
13. Magnesium
14. Manganese
15. Potassium
16. Zinc

What Your Score Means

0-9. Very good. You are reading this book for someone else. (Wouldn't you rather be reading a Tom Clancy novel?)

10-19. You have several sub-clinical or marginal vitamin/mineral deficiencies. (Try not to underline in the book while you are reading or others will know what they are.)

20-32. You have multiple vitamin/mineral deficiencies. (*But you get extra credit if you know what homocysteine is! By the way, homocysteine is a toxic amino acid that can contribute to heart disease.) Taking whole-food supplements can really help you.

To understand where we are, it often helps to know where we came from. Let's look at some history of the American way of eating.

Chapter Two

Who Decided What We Should Eat?

Every culture has roots and traditions, many of which revolve around natural, local foods. For Americans, it's like this. Ask someone what the Basic Four food groups are, and they might reply, "Milk, meat, brownies and ice cream!"

Most guys make grocery shopping quick and easy: They don't usually stop and say, "Hmmm, how many fat grams or calories are in this food?" Like their pre-historic ancestors, they just "grab and run," often returning home with foods they are familiar with such as Oreos or Doritos. Women, on the other hand, shop with a mini-computer, counting every calorie and fat gram, often returning home 15-20 hours later!

Historical Nutrition

When I first began doing research for my nutrition classes in the late seventies, I found an article by Nathaniel Altman entitled, "Nutrition and Watergate: the Story of the Four Food Groups."[6] This article explained that there have been several government-recommended dietary standards throughout the years. I wondered what our other standards were and how they influenced our American health and lifestyles.

The old "Basic Four" Standard American Diet was first introduced in 1956 by the Institute of Home Economics of Agricultural Research of the United States Department of Agriculture (U.S.D.A.) as a standard for good nutrition. However, prior to that time, there was a "Basic Seven" standard and before that one, a "Basic Twelve." Each dietary change was worse, omitting more food groups until it became the "Basic Four." Here is what each dietary group included:

Basic Twelve (1930s)	Basic Seven (1940s)	Basic Four (1956)
1. Milk, dairy prod.	1. Milk, milk products	1. Milk
2. Potatoes, sweet potatoes	2. Tomatoes & fruits	2. Meat
3. Dry peas, beans, nuts	3. Leafy greens	3. Vegetables & fruits
4. Tomatoes & citrus fruits	4. Other vegetables & fruits	4. Breads & cereals
5. Leafy greens & yellow vegetables	5. Butter & fat	
6. Other vegetables and fruits	6. Lean meat, poultry & fish	
7. Eggs	7. Flour & cereals	
8. Lean meat, poultry, fish		
9. Flour and cereals		
10. Butter		
11. Other fat		
12. Sugars		

These standards were designed to help us make healthy choices. In hindsight, the "Basic Twelve" was better because it included many categories of vegetables and fruits and was more balanced than the others. And we now know that butter is healthier than margarine. The "Basic Four" was the worst standard. However, none of these standards were ever based on clinical studies. According to Altman, the meat and dairy industries faced serious financial challenges and through a $30 million campaign they influenced the creation of the "Basic Four."

The American Way

After the "Basic Four" became a national guideline, we saw how these changes damaged our health by reading the results in a Senate Select Committee report published as "The Dietary Goals for the United States," which stated:

The over-consumption of fat, generally, and saturated fat in particular, as well as cholesterol, sugar, salt and alcohol, have been related to six of the ten leading causes of death: heart disease, cancer, cerebrovascular disease, diabetes, arteriosclerosis, and cirrhosis of the liver.[7]

According to doctors and nutritionists consulted, these changes created dietary imbalances which have proven to be damaging to our nation's health. Only within the last twenty years have we begun to understand the dangers of this diet and their link to diabetes, heart disease, and cancer.

An Updated Food Group

It's no wonder that people are still confused. I recently had a client tell me that her idea of a "balanced diet" was a Twinkie in one hand and a soda in the other!

In the mid-1990s, the out-of-date "Basic Four" was replaced by the Eating Right Food Pyramid in an effort to bring balance to our former lopsided dietary guidelines. While this long overdue Food Pyramid was better than the "Basic Four," unfortunately it still needs revision.

The Food Pyramid is a visual representation of how to eat foods relative to each other. For example, it shows that we should get the majority of food we eat from the grain and cereal group. Here is a recap of the Food Pyramid.

Fats and oils: (eat sparingly)
Milk, yogurt and cheese (2-3 servings)
Meat, eggs, poultry, fish, nuts,
    and dry beans (2-3 servings)
Vegetables (3-5 servings)
Fruits (2-4 servings)
Bread, rice, pasta, and cereal (6-11 servings)

Two important changes were: Increase the amount of carbohydrates to more than 6-to-11 servings a day, and decrease the amount of fat from 45 percent to 30 percent. But some vital differences are not clear on the new Food

Pyramid. For example, there is a big difference between a serving of whole-grain bread and processed white bread and between margarine and butter. More importantly, eating so many additional carbohydrates has made our health and weight statistics even worse.

Anyone for Bread or Pasta?

In light of this new standard, with the emphasis on grains and cereals, most of us threw away bacon, eggs and other high-fat foods and began searching for more complex carbohydrates, such as rice and vegetables or pasta for dinner. After all, now we were eating "healthy" foods and getting enough fiber. And carbohydrates were "fat-free." They never told us that excess carbs are also stored in the body as fat!

Being a health nut, I began eating brown rice rather than white rice. My early bean-eating, rice-chewing Macrobiotic days were good. However, after a period of time, I noticed that I didn't feel as good as I used to. Often, I ate toast and cereal for breakfast, whole-wheat sandwiches for lunch, and brown rice and vegetables for dinner. Unfortunately, I gained more weight and couldn't keep it off. In fact, I had worse sugar and carbohydrate cravings than before.

Are You Eating More and Enjoying it Less?

Eating carbohydrates, especially refined and processed carbohydrates such as white bread, white pasta, and refined cereals which turn to sugar, raises insulin. **Insulin is the "fat-storing, hunger-causing" hormone. So eating refined carbohydrates can make you fat!** Additionally, even eating unprocessed carbohydrates, such as wheat bread, brown rice, and high-fiber, whole-grain cereals **can also make you fat,** if you eat too many of them. So the recommended 6 to 11 servings of cereals, grains and pastas hasn't helped us lose weight. On the contrary, it helped us lose our health. Eating excess sugars **and** starches leads to serious problems such as hypoglycemia, diabetes, and many forms of heart disease.

I'm not the only one who has struggled with carbohydrates. The average American eats 250-500 grams of carbohydrates a day (processed breads, cereals, pastas, pizzas, sodas and fruit beverages each contain about 25 or more carbohydrate grams). We used to eat one-third or less of that amount. **Now, nearly half of our population is overweight, and about 13 percent of our children are overweight after following the high-carbohydrate, low-fat way of eating. Clearly, the Food Pyramid isn't healthy.** Yet it's still being taught to school children across the nation, while the incidence of diabetes in children continues to skyrocket.

Whether people are vegetarians or meat-eaters, cutting down on the carbohydrate servings—especially processed carbohydrates—makes people healthier. I recommend only eating 2 to 3 whole-grain carbohydrate servings a day. (For more details, see my first book, *Why Can't I Lose Weight?*)

Have We Lost Control of Our Portions?

Americans eat about 200 calories more per day than they did even fifteen years ago. Americans aren't downsizing! And why should we when we can "super-size" for only 30 cents more!

According to the U.S.D.A, in 1957, the average fast-food soda was 8 ounces and a theatre serving of popcorn was 3 cups. Today, average take-out sodas range from 32-64 ounces and a medium popcorn is 16 cups.

Our dietary standards are lopsided. Our serving sizes are bigger. And we wonder why we are overweight?

Processed Foods

America is an affluent society, blessed with not only natural food, but highly processed foods. In the last ten years, more than ten thousand "convenience processed foods" have been introduced in the United States.

The August 11, 2001 *British Medical Journal* quoted a World Health Organization Report that some of the world's poorest and least developed countries had more efficient healthcare systems than many Western countries. The U.S. ranked 72nd out of 191 countries!

Now What Are We Eating?

Today the average American eats more than 200 pounds of sugar, per person, per year. In the 1880s, people ate less than 12 pounds of sugar, per person, per year.

Today people eat upwards of 55 pounds of fats and oils; more than 300 cans of soft drinks, 50 pounds of cakes and cookies, and 20 gallons of ice cream.[8]

One hundred years ago, heart attacks were practically unheard of in the United States. But a hundred years ago, people ate fresh, whole foods which included meat and butter. However, they didn't eat processed foods. (You'll learn more about processed foods in chapter 5.)

As America was growing stronger economically, she also became a giant in the food-processing industry. As we moved from an agriculture-based society to a high-tech society, our diets, lifestyles, and health profiles have changed.

Among the diseases common among people of countries rich enough to produce processed foods are:

*Heart attacks and strokes *Gallbladder disease
*High blood pressure   *Obesity
*Adult-onset diabetes   *Osteoporosis
And the list could go on and on.

One hundred years ago, we were a much healthier nation. Our American governmental dietary standards have changed dramatically, and not always for the best.

So let's move on to see what effect these dietary changes and processed foods have had on our health.

Chapter Three

Who Decided How Many Vitamins We Need?

When I started studying nutrition nearly twenty-five years ago, I didn't know my magnesium from a gymnasium. I probably had a "B complex" complex! Since that time, I've become fascinated with nutritional therapy and what it can accomplish. But how did it all begin?

A Polish chemist named Casimir Funk first called the anti-beriberi substance in polished rice a "vital amine" which later became "vitamin." Afterwards, Funk and others proposed the "vitamin deficiencies cause disease theory" which said that the absence of one of these vital substances caused disease.

A Popular Example

Today most people have heard about using vitamin C to prevent scurvy. Until Dr. James Lind came along, no one knew the cause of scurvy—a terrible disease that killed tens of thousands of sailors from the 16th to the 18th century.

Scurvy causes an increased weakness of blood vessels, bleeding, and death from massive blood loss. Lind proved that providing sufficient quantities of lime and lemon juice to the sailors could prevent bleeding and blood loss. This is one of the reasons why the British Navy were called "Limeys." Dr. Lind saved thousands of lives by searching for and finding the natural way to prevent and cure scurvy, known as "the sailor's disease."

I have helped hundreds of people with bleeding gums, varicose veins, spider veins, or bruising, by giving them the vitamin C complex from food, not the synthetic counterpart. (You will see that there is a big difference between real vitamin C complex and synthetic ascorbic acid in chapter 7.)

Scurvy is rare today, but it took the British Admiralty more than 40 years to put Dr. Lind's discoveries into practice and distribute limes to British sailors. During those 40 years, thousands of British sailors died needlessly. The world doesn't have to suffer from scurvy anymore, but we do have other serious diseases.

Vitamins Are Powerful

The April 1992 issue of *Time* Magazine was the best-selling issue in the history of the magazine. The cover and title article was "The Real Power of Vitamins," and it looked at the possibility of how vitamins can prevent disease.

Today there are hundreds of thousands of clinical journal articles that show that vitamins and minerals in fruits and vegetables can reduce the risk for a multitude of diseases. They can protect the heart, strengthen the immune system, decrease blood pressure, help manage blood-sugar levels, reduce birth defects, improve brain function, reduce the risk of cancer, improve menstrual cycles, relieve allergies and asthma, protect the bowels, so on. (This list makes me want to take a break and at least eat an organic apple!)

Whether we will get degenerative diseases or not depends on our lifestyle and nutrition. If vitamins are so great, why are we so sick? Often there is a big gap between amount of nutrients in our diet and the amount needed for protection from disease.

Are You Malnourished?

Really, starvation is not just a third-world issue; it's an American lifestyle! While third-world countries don't have enough food, we have plenty of food. The problem is that much of our food has little nutrition.

Nutritional deficiencies can be hard to spot. The food tastes good, looks good, and has calories and energy so we think its okay. The commercial food industry sells billions of dollars of empty "processed" foods. But the term "processed" means something was taken out. Since vital nutrients are missing, even with a full belly we begin to slowly become malnourished.

If it were up to me, I would have made it so much easier to spot nutritional deficiencies. Why not have color-coded disease? For example, if you turn green, you have an eggplant deficiency. If you turn purple, you obviously have a spinach deficiency. And if you turn orange, you need to change your suntan lotion!

The Nutritional Link

Nearly every human health problem has a nutritional component. Here are some examples from my practice:

Bob's high-blood pressure was lowered naturally when I put him on a whole-food supplement called Cardio Plus and changed his diet. His doctor was able to get him off the high-blood pressure medication that he had been taking.

Another client, Janice, had severe fatigue and depression. In three months, she was a different person following my dietary changes and nutrition protocol including folic acid.

Debbie has been a Type 2 diabetic for two years. By making dietary changes and following my nutritional protocol including the B complex and chromium, her blood-sugar levels are now stable and she requires no additional medications.

So many problems or diseases start out as "sub-clinical" or marginal deficiencies that are often ignored or overlooked. These deficiencies are usually not severe enough to produce a real symptom, so they are hard to diagnose. Many of my clients report these symptoms to their doctor who runs several tests, but nothing ever shows up. He's looking for disease. These symptoms are usually linked to nutritional deficiencies years before there is a sign of disease. So their doctor sends them home, telling them to come back when the symptoms are worse. At least then he'll have a drug for the symptoms. But he never addressed the original deficiency.

Can You Get Everything From Food?

In the last chapter, I spoke about the Food Pyramid and stated there was never a clinical trial proving that eating 6-11 servings of carbohydrates would improve the health of the American population. If we ate better, though, could we get everything we need from food? No!

In a similar manner, **there has never been a study of the American diet proving that we get all the vitamins and minerals we need for optimal health through our food.** On the contrary, you can pick up almost any issue of the *American Journal of Clinical Nutrition* and find study after study citing nutritional deficiencies that are linked to heart disease, cancer, diabetes, and so on.

Never before have we eaten so many refined and processed foods with so many missing nutrients. Never before have we been exposed to so many chemicals. And never before have we experienced so much stress.

Grandma Was Healthy

Maybe there was a time when we did get everything from food. One hundred years ago, people lived on farms and people ate their vegetables which were plentiful.

Not today. Some surveys indicate that as many as 59% of our calories come from nutrient-poor foods such as soft drinks, white bread, and snack foods. And as you will learn, our foods don't contain as many nutrients as they once did.

What Were The RDAs?

In 1941, in an attempt to prevent disease, the Food and Nutrition Board of the National Research Council prepared guidelines for vitamins and minerals called the Recommended Dietary Allowances (RDAs). They were originally set up to reduce the rates of serious nutrient-related deaths from diseases such as scurvy, which is a vitamin C deficiency, beriberi, from a lack of thiamine or vitamin B1, and pellagra, a deficiency of niacin, or vitamin B3.

While the RDAs were a step in the right direction, they did not define optimum intake of nutrients. Additionally, they weren't designed for everyone.

Problems with the RDAs

Here are several situations that the RDAs didn't address.

1. They were designed to evaluate the adequacy of the diet of groups of people, not individuals. People vary in their nutritional needs.

2. They did not take into consideration lifestyle and environmental factors which can destroy vitamins. In other words, there was no consideration about the effects of food additives, heavy metals, drugs or alcohol related to nutritional deficiencies.

3. They were amounts for healthy people, so they didn't address the needs of sick people.

4. They didn't account for certain groups: The elderly, pregnant, lactating women, teenagers, smokers, dieters, and people who drink alcohol or take prescription drugs. All of these people need more nutrition than the average person.

5. They were established 50 years ago, before food processing, and increased fast-food consumption.

The old RDAs were never designed to prevent cancer; they just prevented the above-mentioned deficiencies. While we need 10 milligrams of vitamin C to prevent scurvy, we need more than that to prevent heart disease. But it's not easy. A U.S.D.A. government survey of 21,500 people found that not one single person consumed 100% of the RDAs, from the foods they ate.

Another problem with the RDAs is that they are based on 2,000 calories a day. Yet only a certain number of people eat that many calories. And finally, the RDAs **were not established using whole-food vitamin complexes**. For example, the RDAs for vitamin C were established using synthetic ascorbic acid which is only a portion of the entire C complex. But we don't become deficient in just ascorbic acid; we become deficient in the whole complex. As you'll see in chapter 7, only the whole-food complex gives your body the entire nutrition it needs to make up the deficiency. Now people commonly exceed the RDAs with "megadoses." But taking large amounts (1,000 mg.) of a part of the C complex (ascorbic acid), can throw off our body chemistry.

RDIs Replace the RDAs

In 1993, the Nutrition Labeling and Education Act replaced the RDAs with the RDIs (Reference Daily Intake) which represented an average need. The RDAs and RDIs, however, are generally similar values. (I still think it's just another way to confuse us!)

Now you can find the DRV—no, I don't mean your dad's recreational vehicle parked in the driveway! DRV means Daily Recommended Values for Adults, which are the amounts of fats, carbohydrates, fiber, protein, cholesterol, sodium and potassium you should get every day. Finally, the Food and Drug Administration (FDA) has combined the RDIs and DRVs into one standard called the Daily Value (DV). This is the basis for the detailed labels now on food packages. (But the average person still doesn't understand them! More about that in a possible sequel... *Why Can't I Read Food Labels?*)

Most of my clients have taken some vitamins. So on their first visit, they are often confused about whole-food supplements as they relate to them. Their biggest complaint is that they don't see the high number of milligrams on our labels as on other synthetic vitamin labels. But when they return for their follow-up appointment, they are delighted and surprised how well these whole-food supplements work. More about that in chapter 7.

If I Were in Charge...

Personally, I think we should start all over. Here's my three-point proposal:

1. Advertise the benefits of eating fruits and vegetables more. It seems that not getting heart disease or cancer hasn't done the trick. Maybe if we tell people eating fruits and vegetables will make them more money, grow hair on their head, and give them a better sex life, people will eat them!

2. Instead of the RDIs, make a new dietary recommendation: "Recommended Whole Foods Daily Allowances," or RWFDA (for short!) Then we would know exactly what to eat!

3. And while we're at it, I think we should put our national energy in establishing higher standards for better soil, better foods, better restaurants to create better people! (I've found people aren't quite so grumpy when they eat well.)

Obviously, the RDIs aren't changing any time soon, and in the meantime, we still come up short nutritionally. We still need to have an understanding of what we could be missing, and how we can bridge the gaps.

The need for supplements in disease prevention is well documented. Let's look at why.

PART TWO

Why We Really Need Whole-Food Supplements

Chapter Four

Why Do We Need Supplements?

In a perfect world, we should be able to eat healthy meals and never need to take extra supplements. In a perfect world, we should all have thin thighs and buns of steel, too, but that's not going to happen any time soon, either!

Not needing supplements may have been possible in this country 100 years ago before our soils were depleted and before large-scale food processing, but it's not true today. There are simply too many elements that can cause people to become vitamin and mineral deficient.

People Want Results

Most of my clients have become frustrated with traditional drug therapy, and are searching for healthier alternatives. Nutritional supplements are at the top of their lists.

Today, nearly 70% of Americans take some type of vitamins or food supplements. More than 3,000 vitamin and mineral supplements stand on shelves in health food stores around the country. The supplement industry is a more than $16 billion a year industry.

More Than Genetics

Although it is true that genetics play a role in our health profile, a disease that runs in a family is not always genetically related. Often, everyone in a family eats the same nutrient-depleted diet and follows the same sedentary lifestyle. Often we get what mom or dad got because we eat like they ate! Our health and protection from disease depends on many factors, and a large one is supplementation. Let's begin by looking at five reasons you may need to supplement your diet.

1. To Makeup for Our Unhealthy Lifestyles

Nutrient deficiencies created by our American diet can cause the body to be prone to a number of symptoms including viruses, infections, allergies, headaches, fatigue, bowel problems, heart attacks, and arthritis.

The 1997 World Health Report stated that our modern diet is too high in fat, sugar, sodium, and saturated fat, and it doesn't provide enough vitamins, minerals or fiber to meet our nutritional needs. The sad fact is that **anywhere people have adopted our American diet, there has been an increase in heart disease, strokes and cancers.** Uh-oh!

Even at our best, who has the time, energy and money to eat a "well-balanced" diet every day? Even if we **could** get all the nutrition from our diets, only 9% of the population eats the recommended five to nine servings of protective fruits and vegetables. And God knows how many parents have tried to make their children eat asparagus!

During an interview with Dr. Joel Robbins, from the Health and Wellness Center in Tulsa, Oklahoma, he gave three reasons for using food supplements in his practice.

1. The average person can't change their diet to a more nutritious lifestyle overnight. These changes take time. In the meantime, they should supplement their diet.

2. Digestive problems that were developed **prior** to changing their diet to a more healthful lifestyle **will hinder full assimilation** of the nutrients in the healthy foods they consume. So they need extra nutrition to make up for these deficiencies.

3. There is a **limit** to what the body can assimilate in a day. We can't assimilate enough carrots in a day, to make up for a long-standing vitamin A deficiency. We need supplements.

Taking supplements bridges the gap between what you would like to eat and what you actually eat. It can take a long time between the depletion of vitamin stores in our body and the full-blown deficiency symptoms to manifest. Clinical nutritionist Shari Lieberman says, "It is not until the depletion is prolonged and severe that the classic clinical signs of deficiency appear."[9] By then it's often advanced, and the person requires several supplements over a longer period.

In other words, even if we consume a totally perfect diet, it cannot contain enough nutrition to take care of today's needs **and** have enough left over for **paying back long-standing nutritional deficiencies.** That's why I highly recommend whole-food supplements to the majority of my clients for at least a three-to-six month period or even years to improve severe or multiple deficiencies.

You Need Supplements If...

Our lifestyles and habits prevent us from getting the nutrition we need. Our American lifestyle of eating sugar, drinking caffeine, or drinking alcohol, at least hinders absorption of minerals, and at worst, further aggravates a mineral deficiency. For example, a calcium deficiency is commonly linked to excess of caffeine from any source.

Even health-minded clients need help. Jean, in her quest to be healthier, avoided all red meat and dairy, but she took no supplements. Through biochemical nutritional testing, I found she was deficient in protein, zinc, the entire B complex, calcium and several minerals. It took her four months to regrow her hair and regain her strength.

Here are some other factors that increase the amounts of nutrients we need. Nearly every one of these depletes water-soluble vitamins and several minerals.

41

You Need Supplements If You Are...

*Drinking coffee and tea	*Pregnant
*Eating processed/overcooked foods	*Taking laxatives
*Experiencing poor digestion	*Drinking alcohol
*Using medical drugs	*Feeling depressed
*Experiencing illness	*Following fad diets
*Regularly using oral contraceptives	*Exercising excessively
*Recovering from a cold or surgery	*Experiencing PMS
*Living a stressful lifestyle	*Experiencing food allergies
*Not getting fruits & vegetables	*Smoking
*Being exposed to radiation/pollution	*Struggling with diabetes

If you can identify even five out of the above list, you probably are marginally deficient in several vitamins and minerals and would benefit from whole-food supplements.

Not only is the average diet deficient in vitamins and minerals, it's highly **toxic.** (See chapter 5.) This requires the body to use the vitamins and minerals it gets to neutralize the toxins so they don't kill us. Where can the body get these nutrients if we don't take extra supplements?

Many Americans take some type of pharmaceutical drug. Many drugs interact with nutrients in the body, often causing further depletion. **For example, taking the birth control pill depletes your levels of vitamin C, B and E. Antacids commonly hinder the absorption of calcium.**

Supplements are not a substitute for a healthy diet, but taking supplements is good insurance. At least you will be getting the minimal amounts required to keep you healthy.

2. To Replenish What's Missing in our Soil.

One hundred years ago, all of our soil was "organic." People were healthier, too.

I've already mentioned that the average American doesn't even eat their recommended servings of fruits and vegetables.

The sad part is that the fruits and vegetables they do grab are frighteningly low in minerals. **For example, the most popular vegetable eaten by teens is French fries!**

Minerals are essential for our health and longevity. Everyone knows that we need calcium for healthy bones and teeth or iron to prevent iron-deficiency anemia. We need both macro and trace minerals. Our body can produce some vitamins, but it can't produce minerals. Vegetables absorb minerals from the soil, so we depend on them as sources for minerals. **But what if these valuable minerals aren't in the soil? Then we need to take them as a supplement.**

There is a great link between mineral-deficient soil and disease, which increases the vital need for at least whole-food mineral supplementation.

Unfortunately, our soils are depleted because of the use of chemical fertilizers. Dr. Elson Haas, in *Staying Healthy With Nutrition* says:

> ...fertilizers can create some imbalances in the soil and produce depletion of other important minerals, such as chromium, selenium, and iodine. Heavy metals such as lead and mercury can also contaminate soil.[10]

Chromium, for example, is a trace mineral required to help maintain normal blood-sugar levels, but because of the use of commercial fertilizers it's often either not in our soil, or it's hard to assimilate. That's why chromium is such a common deficiency throughout the United States.

Dr. Don Colbert in *What You Don't Know May Be Killing You* stated: "Without question, I believe that mineral deficiency is a major factor in the increased levels of disease in the United States."[11]

In 1948, you could buy spinach that contained 158 milligrams of iron. Today, the iron content of raw spinach is 27 milligrams. That means you would have to eat 6 bowls of spinach to get the same amount of iron that one bowl might have given you back in 1948.[12]

I'll give more details about our soil and deficiencies in chapter 6, but the best way to make up deficiencies is not only to eat organically grown fruits and vegetables, but also to take supplements grown in truly organic soil. (I'll discuss how to identify whole-food supplements in part 3.)

3. To Replenish What's Missing in Our Food

Unfortunately, we can't depend on our food supply to give our bodies enough nutrition for optimum health. Few people grow their own organic food and eat it fresh. We'll look further at how the food is grown in chapter 6, but what about the processing and handling of our food?

Foods are usually transported across the country for days before they get to the supermarket, losing precious vitamins and minerals from exposure to light and air.

Food-processing, which includes canning and preserving destroys essential nutrients. For example, there is little or no folic acid left in canned vegetables. Folic acid in a pregnant women's diet will prevent spina bifida, but it also helps prevent depression, cervical dysplasia and colon cancer.

Cooking food reduces its nutritional value by destroying 20% to 50% of vitamins, all enzymes, and many minerals. Boiling vegetables destroys most folic acid and vitamin C. Milling whole grains to make white flour results in 70% loss of vitamins, minerals and fiber. Even broiling meat destroys one-third of the B1 vitamin, thiamine.

Even if you ate your recommended portions of produce, it's highly unlikely that you are getting **all** of the vitamins and minerals required for optimal health. By supplementing your diet, you can replenish what is missing in your food.

4. To Help You Deal With Stressors

The Environmental Protection Agency (EPA) estimates that 60,000 chemicals have been buried or dumped throughout the U.S. over the last hundred years. There are over 3,000 different carcinogenic chemicals in our foods. Foreign to your body, these chemicals attack your cells in a process that leads to disease.

In addition, pollution and the depletion of the ozone layer create free radicals which attack your cells. More than 80 diseases have been linked to free radical damage. Our bodies don't make enough antioxidants to combat the damaging effects of environmental pollution.

And everybody feels the demands of life and stress. It seems that even children and teenagers need "Daytimers" to schedule all of their activities! Toddlers may never need a "Daytimer" but think about the stress their tiny bodies go through running around with Mommy all day—eating Lunchables or chicken nuggets! Stress depletes crucial nutrients, especially the water-soluble B and C vitamins, and a host of minerals.

Additionally, even good stress, such as regular aerobic exercise can increase your nutrient requirements. The increased needs are not met by the standard American diet, but can only be met with additional supplementation.

5. To Prevent or Reverse Disease

So often clients return to see me on their two-week follow-up and say, "I've changed my diet! I'm not eating any sugar or white-flour products. I'm eating lots of fruits and vegetables now. So now can I get off these supplements?"

Even if you eat a nutrient-dense diet from today forward, what about the still-present nutritional deficiencies which took years to develop? What about the last 10 or 20 years of consuming a poor diet?

The body uses nutrition first for day-to-day survival. Healing is the body's second priority. **It's only when nutrients are left over at the end of the day that the body can heal. That's why natural healing takes time. We have** to continue to feed small amounts of whole foods over a period of months, or even years in the case of severe deficiency and disease, to help the body return to health.

Build Your Immune System

Most diseases weaken our immune system. It's easy to "get behind" in our nutrition which lowers our immunity.

A client named Candy came to see me with severe fibromyalgia. She followed my nutritional protocol of supplements including: Flaxseed oil, a B vitamin complex, magnesium, antioxidant vitamins, digestive enzymes and a multiple vitamin. Within days she felt better and in three months, she was able to work in her garden and do housework without any pain. She's still doing well.

What about serious diseases such as cancer? Nutritionist Dr. Patrick Quillin says that one of the primary causes of cancer is poor nutrition: An excess, deficiency, or imbalance of any nutrient. Additionally, here are three reasons why he uses nutrition in cancer treatment:

1. **To avoid malnutrition.** Forty percent or more of cancer patients actually die from malnutrition, not from cancer.

2. **To reduce the toxic effects of chemo and radiation.** He explains that properly nourished patients experience less nausea, malaise, immune suppression, hair loss, and organ toxicity than patients on routine oncology programs.

3. **To bolster immune functions.** There is an abundance of data linking nutrient intake to the quality and quantity of immune factors that fight cancer.[13]

We need supplements to make up nutritional deficiencies in our diet and lifestyles, to make up missing nutrients in our soil, to make up for lost nutrients in the handling of our food, to help us deal with stressors, and to prevent serious disease.

Only whole-food supplements made from real food combined with healthy lifestyle can truly make up for these nutritional deficiencies.

Chapter Five

Is Our Food Really Food?

Processed foods have been around for a long time, but eating fast foods wasn't God's idea. I can't imagine Adam and Eve looking for Twinkies or Ding Dongs. Besides, we all know they much preferred apples!

Processed foods are everywhere. Lisa Messinger, author of *Why Should I Eat Better?* says: "There is $400 billion floating around out there trying to get you to eat processed food, which is the largest industry in the United States."[14]

And we do. The average American now eats 200 pounds of sugar per person per year. And yet we still wonder why we are tired, or why we can't lose weight!

Who Taught You To Eat?

Most of us eat like our parents ate, and they ate like their parents ate. Well, who taught them? We have all been influenced by the governmental food guidelines, but a great deal of our nutritional education came from media advertising. Here's an example. Things go better with a what? Most people in America of all ages would answer, "Coke."

But just because it's on TV doesn't mean it's good for you. In their book, *Empty Harvest,* the authors reprinted a cigarette advertisement from 1937 that claimed "Camel cigarettes help digest food." Another sugar advertisement they reprinted said, "Science shows how sugar can help keep your appetite—and weight—under control." **This ad actually tries to convince you that you need refined, white sugar in your diet!**[15]

It makes you wonder how we knew what to eat before television commercials and newspaper advertisements!

Can Man Make Food Better Than God?

Compare a natural food, such as an apple, to a man-made food such as a donut. Apples are rich in nutrients, water and fiber, while the donut is made from white sugar, white flour, and hydrogenated fats. Not only does the donut contain sugar and fat—it doesn't have much nutrition. So it can deplete your own store of vitamins, minerals and enzymes.

But when was the last time you stopped at the grocery store to buy a dozen apples to take to work rather than donuts?

As with most man-made products, refined and processed foods are so different from their original form that our bodies do not even recognize them as a food but rather a food substitute.

What Are Teens Eating?

Burgess Parks, husband of nutrition author Mary June Parks, spent 32 years as a public school administrator. When he retired in 1970, there were only isolated cases of teachers being attacked. Today violence in schools is rampant. But no one asks about their diets. When they check the diets of juvenile delinquents, they are filled with sugar-laden junk food.[16]

It's no wonder violent behavior is increasing—since high amounts of sugar and soda cause B vitamin deficiencies. Symptoms of a serious B vitamin deficiency include: anxiety, depression, mental confusion, insanity, irritability, and rage.

According to Mary June, many diseases are related to sugar consumption: Allergies, arthritis, asthma, cancer, cataracts, constipation, epilepsy, fatigue, heart disease, hyperactivity in adults and children, depression, headaches, sinus trouble, tooth decay, hypoglycemia, mental illness, memory loss, migraines, varicose veins, diabetes and PMS.[17]

Sugar in Foods

I think foods should be defined by what they do to your body. How about, "diabetes-inducing white sugar," or "artery-clogging margarine?" No longer will you think of these as "Foods I can't have." Soon you will be describing them as "Foods I don't want!"

No one would intentionally sit down and eat several teaspoons of sugar at once. But they add up. The number of teaspoons of sugar in some foods can range from 5 to 15. You may not think you eat sugar, but it's found in nearly everything: Salad dressings, ketchup, mayonnaise, peanut butter, soups, pickles, cereals, canned fruits, luncheon meats, crackers, breads and juices.

So you may have decided to switch to sugar substitutes. Many other countries have banned artificial sweeteners because of their link to cancer risk.

Additionally, refined white flour foods such as white bread and pasta, turn to sugar in the liver. So not only does sugar cause deficiencies, but white flour products do as well.

The Whole Grain and Nothing but the Grain

Even as far back as 1942, a nutrition-minded dentist named Dr. Royal Lee was calling for legislative action to protect the public health when he said:

> No food is safe unless it is fresh enough to retain its perishable vitamins, incurred no processing that would remove or impair its vitamin and mineral content; free of any kind of synthetic adulteration, and unless it has a background of experience behind it establishing its value to the human family.[18]

Did you know that up to 70 percent of the essential nutrients are lost in the production of white flour? After white flour is rolled, it's then bleached by chlorine dioxide where any vitamin E is completely destroyed. In the refinement process, more than 21 nutrients are taken out, and only a handful are put back in.

There is so much evidence of the correlation between heart disease and white flour that Dr. Lee said, **"We might as well remove the term heart disease and supplant it with 'white-flour disease.'"**[19]

Dr. Lee said that a better way to make flour is to grind it with stone buhrs to as fine a degree as possible; then sift out the major part of the fibrous remainder. This retains the complete germ portion of the wheat. Of course, he added that since this flour requires refrigeration, manufacturers would have to use vacuum-packed tins.[20]

In chapter 2, I mentioned that eating too many carbohydrates makes us fat. But it does more than that. High insulin levels increase the cell's cholesterol-making ability. So eating processed carbs puts us at risk for even greater problems such as high cholesterol, diabetes, heart disease, chronic fatigue, accelerated aging, arthritis, and even cancer.

We Need the Good Stuff

Dr. Lee said it well:

America's food industry is built to a large extent on foods which would ordinarily be highly perishable. Rather than finding methods of efficient distribution, it has been easier to simply devitalize the food. Foods which have had their vital factors removed will fail to sustain life for insects, molds, and microbes; consequently they can be easily shipped over long distances, and simply stored over long periods. Unfortunately foods which will not sustain other forms of life, will not satisfactorily sustain human life.[21]

This reminds me of M&M's. Ants ignore them on a picnic—they go for your chicken sandwich! We should be smarter than ants!

You can read more about the harmful effect of sugar and starches in my book, *Why Can't I Lose Weight?* The rest of this chapter will focus on the processing and types of fat.

What About Cholesterol and Diet?

We're born with a desire to eat and enjoy good fat. I didn't always know that. In fact, I've tried "no-fat" diets, and it was hard to eat bread without butter or eat salad without salad dressing. After a few days, I searched for the most fatty foods I could find. Going no-fat was no fun!

For many years, I read articles about how butter was a "saturated" fat and we shouldn't eat it if we were trying to lose weight, or if we had high cholesterol.

But did you know that eighty percent of cholesterol is produced by the body itself? The way to lower cholesterol levels is not to restrict dietary cholesterol, but reduce the mechanism by which cholesterol is made. The best way to do this is to eat a diet low in sugars and processed carbohydrates.

Butter Is Better!

Dr. Royal Lee considered raw, unpasteurized butter to be one of the highest values in food products obtainable. In one of his reports, he wrote, "Butter is rich in vitamins A, D, E and F. Taken the year round, butter contains enough vitamin D to be considered a preferred source of this vitamin."[22]

In this same report, Dr. Lee even quoted a study that simply used butter to treat psoriasis, xerophthalmia [a skin disease], tuberculosis, dental caries and rickets![23]

He also said that substituting vegetable oils for butter caused a decalcification of bones, resulting in their fragility, which he believed was a vitamin F deficiency.[24]

51

In another story, Dr. Lee reported that during World War One, Denmark exported most of its butter and replaced it with butter substitutes. The result was a tragically high incidence of children becoming blind.[25]

Omega 3 Fats Are Essential

Everyone is familiar with the term essential amino acid. This means there are certain amino acids that our body doesn't make, that we must obtain from outside sources—our diet. The same is true of fats. Some fats are essential because they are not made by the body, but are required by food or supplementation.

Most Americans get enough Omega 6 and 9 fats from foods like butter and animal products. But they are deficient in the Omega 3 fats. Examples of these fats are flaxseeds, walnuts, Salmon, tuna, and other cold-water fish.

Are You Craving Fats or Sugar?

We desperately need some good fat! When your body is fat-starved, you get hungry, overeat, and binge on carbohydrates and sweets. Many people think they have a "sweet tooth," when in fact, they may have a "fat tooth." Often what they really want when they think they want sweets is fat. For example, people crave chewy cookies, flavored yogurt, and double-chocolate ice cream. The first ingredient in the label may be **sugar,** but the second ingredient is **fat.**

We're All Deficient

All of us are deficient in the good types of fats because the typical American diet doesn't include them. What we are experiencing in America is a major essential fatty acid (EFA) deficiency.

Scientist Brian Peskin in his book, *Beyond the Zone,* said:

In the 1930s, Americans switched from eating butter and other natural fats and oils to highly refined unsaturated oils, margarine and hydrogenated shortening. That's when the high rate of heart disease increased.[26]

Good fats are vital for health. Here's a list of what the Omega 3 fats can do for the body (taken from my book, *Why Can't I Lose Weight?*):

*Boost the immune system

*Carry and store fat-soluble vitamins A, D, E, K (for skin and blood clotting)

*Are necessary to make healthy hair, skin, and nails

*Are required to build hormones to assist in the treatment and prevention of PMS and other hormonal problems

*Are an excellent source of energy

*Reduce food cravings and help you feel satisfied

*Can lower cholesterol and triglycerides[27]

Another Great Fat

Olive oil has been a staple for 5,000 years. Populations who use olive oil have a much lower incidence of heart disease and strokes. One reason is that olive oil is the richest monounsaturated fat, and it lowers the bad (LDL) cholesterol.

Refined oils, on the other hand, are quite different from the original product. Refinement means that the oil is clear, odorless, and almost completely devoid of nutrients.

Trans Fats Are Damaged Fats

"Trans fats" are fats that have been altered or damaged by high heat. These are a man-made type of fat not found naturally. Processors hydrogenate or add hydrogen molecules to vegetable oils under high heat. What would normally be a liquid oil now becomes solid at room temperature. A good example is margarine.

These trans-fatty acids not only raise the bad LDL cholesterol level, just like saturated fat, but they also lower the good HDL cholesterol. They hinder your body's ability to use the fat-soluble vitamins, they add to the load of our already overworked liver, and they even cause an essential fatty acid deficiency. What's worse, they hinder weight loss.

Obviously, as Scientist Brian Peskin says, trans fats are linked to heart disease.

> Trans-unsaturated fat, as the man-made stuff is called, is 14 times more potent as a disease risk factor than the saturated fats the public has been warned about for years—the kind in marbled beef, butter, and cheese.[28]

Since our heart problems are linked to an increase in trans fats and a deficiency in essential fats, a better and safer approach is to dump the trans fats and start taking these essential fats and small amounts of raw butter.

Where Do You Get Trans Fats?

Trans or damaged fats are found in margarine, shortening, mayonnaise, and baked goods containing hydrogenated oils and are commonly called "hydrogenated" or "partially hydrogenated" fats. These include breads, cookies, cakes, potato chips, corn chips, taco shells, all commercial vegetable oils, commercial peanut butter, and all fried foods.

Margarine, shortening, and spread blends are all hydrogenated. Studies have shown that margarine actually coats the stomach wall, rendering foods indigestible. Examples of these are anything that starts with "I can't believe it's...." (I can't believe that people are still eating these foods!)

Unfortunately, most restaurants use either processed heat-treated vegetable oils or hydrogenated vegetable margarine or both. To add insult to injury, they heat them over and over.

What About Fake Fats?

Fat substitutes like Olestra are available. The label contains warnings about possible digestion problems saying that it may inhibit the absorption of vitamins, and recommends using it in moderation. You may have heard that it can cause "anal leakage." Does this sound normal or healthy? (If we **could** eat everything in moderation, we wouldn't need fat substitutes!)

I've helped women lose weight by eating more good fat, not eliminating it or eating fat substitutes. When it comes to food and health, we're better off eating foods as close to their natural state as possible.

Food Preservation

Food used to be preserved naturally somewhat like our grandparents preserved food with salt and vinegar. That way, they could store food from one season to another. Today, the main reason food processors preserve food is to gain a longer shelf life.

In fact, some processed foods will stay on the shelves longer than Americans will stay on the planet!

The average American eats about six pounds of chemicals a year. Three thousand chemicals are added to our foods daily. These chemicals are "man-made" in a laboratory and are foreign to our bodies. Instead of adding health and vitality, they are causing a greater burden on the immune system and filter systems. Additionally, no one has ever studied the cumulative effect of all of these food additives and preservatives on our bodies. We assume the FDA is looking out for us, but they don't have the time or resources to test the thousands of additives on the market.

How Should We Eat?

How do we know what to eat? It's simple: Real food heals. Chemically-based food doesn't. An article in the *Journal of the American Medical Association* showed that people who eat at least five servings of fruits and vegetables a day have a 31% lower risk of stroke than those who eat less than three servings.[29]

Wouldn't it be great if you were required to show your blood reports before ordering at restaurants? Or, you had to pay extra for foods such as French fries or deep fried onion rings? But now my love for science fiction is taking over. Back to reality.

Around the world, there are many other cultures healthier than us. People living along the Mediterranean Sea, for example, have lower rates of colon cancer, breast cancer and coronary heart disease. Their diet consists of fruits and vegetables, beans, nuts and seeds, olive oil, dark bread, pasta, whole grains, cheese, yogurt, fish, eggs and lean meat. What do these foods have in common? They are long-lived, whole, natural foods, all considered to be nutrient dense. (See Food Source of Vitamins in the Appendix on page 101.)

Yes, I know it's hard to find natural, unprocessed foods, plan meals, shop and prepare good food. (You might think that only health food nuts and Oprah Winfrey can eat like this!) I tell my clients to do the best they can, but I also highly recommend that they take organically-grown food supplements to make up for the nutritional deficiencies.

So many of my clients have asked me about organically-grown foods, that I wrote a whole chapter about the soil, and why organic foods are so much better for us. Let's move on to chapter 6.

Chapter Six

Does Our Soil Grow Healthy Food?

If we interviewed the soil that probably grew the food that you ate today, what would it say? I imagine it would go something like this: "I feel so tired; I constantly have a low-grade infection, and I desperately need some rest!"

In chapter 4, one reason I gave for needing supplements is to replenish what's missing in our soil. Few people grow their own gardens anymore. We are so removed from growing our own food, that we just assume the soil is healthy. But is it? Soil is a living thing, too; and like you, it can be weak or sick making it unable to grow healthy foods.

Vegetables Without Vitamins?

We can't expect to live long and healthy lives if we keep eating food grown on malnourished soil. So you might be wondering how nutritious is our soil?

In an article in *Life Extension Magazine* about the nutritional decline of foods from 1963 to 1975, the authors compared the nutrient values for a dozen fruits and vegetables and found that the nutrient value of many foods had dropped significantly. **The amount of vitamin C in sweet peppers dropped from 128 to 89 mg. The vitamin A in collards dropped from 6,500 I.U. to 3,800 I.U.**[30]

That article also stated that The National Academy of Sciences issued an alert saying that **it takes twice as many vegetables to get the daily requirement of vitamin A as previously thought.** The U.S.D.A. was asked if they would have to double the required servings of vegetables in the Food Pyramid to make up for the vitamins lost. No changes were made, and their response was **"The nutritional content of produce is not as important as things like appearance and big yield."**[31] Clearly, you can't depend on the government to protect you when it comes to getting adequate nutrition!

Vegetables are a major source of nutrition. **Without enough folic acid, for example, we put ourselves at risk for heart disease and colon cancer. Without adequate vitamins C and E, we are at risk for other cancers.** Without zinc, there can be an eating disorder. I've helped many clients with eating disorders, and the most important part of the protocol is zinc. We are missing vital nutrients and phytonutrients which are putting us at risk for serious disease.

Earlier in this book, I said that only 9% of Americans get their 5 servings of fruits and vegetables. **If people aren't even eating their vegetables, how are they getting their vitamins? They aren't!** Unfortunately, the vegetables they do eat probably don't contain much nutrition.

What can we do? We must take supplements, but more importantly, we must take whole-food supplements (see chapter 7), grown on organic soil.

Why Organic?

Organic refers to "environmentally friendly" farming methods. In his healthy shopping guide, Dr. Elson Haas lists several natural farming methods including: Developing healthy soil through natural composting; using crop rotation to rest the soil; using intercrop planting; using cover crops to secure the soil against erosion; healthy cultivation practices; controlling pests with natural means; diversifying crops and agriculture methods; and using natural enemies of harmful insects such as spiders and ladybugs.[32]

Here are three reasons why I encourage my clients to buy organic fruits and vegetables, or at least purchase whole-food supplements that are organically-grown.

1. **Organically grown foods are far more nutrient dense.** Sue Frederick gives two good studies in her book, *How To Shop a Natural Foods Store...and Why:*

> Ounce for ounce, organic fruits and vegetables are twice as rich in some nutrients as comparable commercial products, according to a recent study reported in *The Journal of Applied Nutrition.*...commercial fruits and vegetables aren't as good as they used to be. [33]

> Other studies found that vine-ripened organic tomatoes contain twice as much vitamin C than tomatoes that are picked green and artificially ripened with chemicals. [34]

In his book, Dr. Haas quotes these studies:

> A Danish study found that men who consumed a diet composed of at least 25% organic produce had sperm counts 43% higher than those who ate conventional foods. [35]

> Another study found that on average, organic pears, apples, potatoes, sweet corn, and wheat had over 90% more vitamins and minerals than similar commercial food—almost twice the nutrient content. [36]

Wow! Some of these studies might make you want to grow your own food. Like that's going to happen—most people don't even have time to eat food, much less grow it!

2. **Organically grown foods don't contain harmful synthetic chemicals.** The pesticides used by organic farmers break down into harmless ingredients. Organic farmers rotate their crops because this makes them less vulnerable to pests naturally. Dr. Haas says that chemical warfare has gotten out of hand:

> In 1995, the United States alone used 270 billion pounds of artificial fertilizers and 2 billion pounds of pesticides. For the

last twenty years, the U.S. agricultural industry has used more than 1 billion pounds of pesticides annually.[37]

Sue Frederick reports that: "More than 20,000 pesticides are registered for use in the United States."[38] While these pesticides are toxic to pests, they are also toxic to people. She also reports that according to the World Health Organization (WHO), about 25 million people are poisoned by farm chemicals every year. The Environmental Protection Agency (EPA) considers 60% of all herbicides, 90% of all fungicides and 30% of all insecticides carcinogenic. In 1987, a report entitled, "Regulating Pesticides in Food" estimated that pesticide use is linked to 20,000 cases of cancer yearly.[39]

Scary, isn't it? Yet we don't have a clue about the soil that is growing the food we eat every day.

3. **Organic farmers naturally replenish the soil.** The organic farmer studies the soil composition through various tests and replenishes the soil naturally. They use natural fertilizers and rich compost such as manure and fish emulsions to build up the soil and to enhance growth and create a balance of natural nutrients and minerals.

Today's Farming

What happens when the non-organic, commercial farmer spots disease on his plant? He buys dozens of chemicals to treat the plant.

I grew an "organic" garden for three years when I lived in Spokane, Washington. Our fruits and vegetables were so healthy, we didn't have to fight aphids, we just had to keep the birds and dogs away from our harvest! If we treat our soil right, the plants will be healthy!

Fertilized to Death?

In his book, *A Cancer Therapy,* Dr. Max Gerson said:

The damage that modern civilization brings into our lives begins with the soil, where artificial fertilization leads to the displacement of mineral contents and changes in the flora of microbes combined with the exodus of the earthworms.[40]

Dr. Gerson is saying here that there are several major problems with modern farming methods. Chemical fertilizers damage the soil, they cause unbalanced mineral content, they cause an unbalance of vital flora and the loss of precious earthworms.

The soil needs earthworms. When I was a young girl growing up in the country in New York, after a heavy rain we would go outside and get earthworms for fishing bait. These worms are a sign of healthy soil; their presence keeps the soil from getting compacted and keeps it fertile.

Plants grown on land which has been treated poorly are sick. No wonder the farmer needs poisons to kill insects. If he would have taken care of the soil, he would have healthier plants, and his need for insecticides would be greatly reduced.

Unfortunately, there's a big difference between soil fertilized naturally and soil fertilized with chemical fertilizers, and we pay the price with deficient plants and diseased people.

Since 1945, farmers began using chemical fertilizers. But these harsh chemicals stay in the soil for years. California, one of the most progressive of the states, has strict laws for selling organic produce. But it takes time. Crops can't be certified organic unless no chemicals have been used for at least three years.

So What Can You Do?

At the very least, buy organic food as much as you can, and supplement your diet with whole-food supplements which are organically grown. You'll learn more about these next.

Let's now look at the differences in the quality of vitamin supplements.

PART THREE

How To Buy and Take Supplements

Chapter Seven

Are All Supplements Alike?

Purchasing supplements has become a real science, even for women who are born licensed and certified shoppers!

Buying shoes is much easier: Find the right color, size and fit—that's it. Take them to the counter and pay for them. Buying supplements is complicated. One of the last times I bought vitamin C at a health food store, I felt overwhelmed at the possibilities: Should I get the buffered, esterfied, or with bioflavonoids? Should I get liquid, capsules or tablets?

Yet we need supplements. **We can't eat enough food to obtain the disease-preventing or disease-treating benefits of most supplements.** For example, we would have to eat 2 quarts of corn oil, 5 pounds of wheat germ, 8 cups of almonds, or 28 cups of peanuts in order to consume 400 international units of vitamin E.[41]

What's the Difference?

When I teach weight-loss workshops, I hear all kinds of stories about supplements that work and some that don't. For example, one woman told me about her experiences taking a high-powered herbal supplement. She was happy with the weight loss; the downside was that she was often up until 3:00 a.m. wanting to do something invigorating—like washing and waxing her car!

I tell my clients to be wary of vitamins with names like "A Buncha Vitamins," or "Almost All the Vitamins You Probably Need!" And you'll know if you're being ripped off if you buy supplements in "three easy payments."

You may be like so many of my clients who have a cabinet full of a variety of supplements and vitamins, but you still don't feel any better.

My clients often tell me they have taken some type of vitamin for a period of time and either it never worked or it worked at first and then stopped "working." I wondered why? This doesn't happen with food. Does the nutrition in an orange stop working? No. Does the nutrition in an apple or a carrot stop working? No.

To answer the question of whether vitamins work or not we need to look at the type of supplement and how the body uses them. **This is known as "bioavailability," or how they are available to the cells, which all depends on the source.**

Types of Supplements

Early in my practice, I discovered that I could contact several manufactureres and put my own "private label" on a vitamin to sell. That's why in stores, vitamin C can be sold under 10 to 20 different labels, but most of it is the same stuff, produced by just a handful of manufacturing companies.

Most supplements aren't regulated by the FDA. As Judith DeCava reports, "...the nutrition industry has turned into a money-grabbing, hustling, lying, cheating scam." Her research shows that only 3 percent of nutrition companies manufacture their own product! Other companies slap on a private label which frequently contains incorrect information.[42] Just a few large drug companies such as Merck and Hoffman-LaRoche produce the synthetic vitamins used in the rest of the nutritional supplements found in drug stores, health food stores and even doctor's offices.[43]

So what's the difference between these supplements? I recently interviewed Dr. Joel Robbins who teaches a class about natural supplementation. According to Dr. Robbins, there are only **three types of supplements** on the market today. Only one is a true food supplement; the other two are man-made.

Whole-Food Supplements

Whole-food supplements are whole foods with only the water and fiber removed; in other words, they are dried food. They are processed below 112° F. so the enzymes are alive, and they have a limited shelf life. They contain **all** of the nutrients required by our body to meet the needs of our cells.

Synthetic Vitamins

Synthetic vitamins don't come from food. For example, ascorbic acid comes from corn sugar to make vitamin C. Thiamine comes from petroleum or coal tar products to make vitamin B. Eastman Kodak Company supplies almost all supplement companies with synthetic alpha-tocopherol made from distilled cottonseed oil to make vitamin E.[44]

Most drugstore vitamins are synthetic. While they are the exact molecular formula of the organic nutrient, they contain **none of the co-factors required for your body to use this vitamin!** This process causes it to become a "mirror image" of the natural counterpart. Chemically, it has the opposite configuration (left-hand spin instead of right hand spin), so the vitamin can't be used. According to Dr. Gilbert Levin:

> Because its structure is reversed, a left-handed molecule cannot take part in chemical reactions meant for a right-handed molecule any more than a left hand can fit in a right-handed glove: its odd geometry would prevent it from being metabolized by the body. [45]

According to Dr. Lee, not only are these vitamins not usable by the body, but the required co-factors are taken from your own body's reserves, so you become nutritionally deficient.[46]

Crystalline Vitamins

Dr. Robbins teaches that the third type is **crystalline vitamins or fractionated vitamins which are made by treating natural foods with high-powered chemicals, solvents, and heat.** This process destroys **almost all** of the co-factors (enzymes, antioxidants, trace elements and other unknown factors) that are needed for your body to use the vitamin. This can cause vitamin deficiencies.

While this process keeps the right-hand spin, it contains only **part** of the real thing like comparing refined white flour (crystalline vitamin) to wheat flour (whole-food supplement). You miss the major ingredients. According to Dr. Robbins, the motivation for producing crystalline vitamins is to increase the milligram levels for marketing purposes only, not for our good health.

Problems With Vitamins That Are Not Whole-Food Supplements

According to Dr. Robbins, there are many problems with synthetic vitamins.

1. The first problem is that synthetic vitamins create nutritional deficiencies.

2. Another problem is that synthetic vitamins don't just pass through the body; the body has to process them. Since they are processed by the body, they can be harmful. (See chapter 8.)

3. A third problem is that rather than work as a true nutrient, they work as a stimulant. That's why you often experience a "rush" when taking synthetic vitamins.

4. A fourth problem is freshness. The FDA does not require expiration dates on vitamins, so many companies don't include them. **Calcium supplements can sit on the shelf for years before you purchase them.** If they don't have an expiration date, they are packed with preservatives. Whole-food supplements have a dated shelf-life.

What's on the label isn't always what's in the pill! And there are many misleading labels. Let's look at some common examples.

Labeling Deceptions

You'll see the word, "natural," written on everything these days. **Did you know that most vitamins on the market claiming to be natural only have to be 10% natural to make this claim?**

Here's an example from a flyer on vitamin E. "Some firms mix 10% natural vitamin E with 90% synthetic vitamin E and call their product "natural" vitamin E without declaring the synthetic portion. The Food and Drug Administration (FDA) has yet to act to stop this misleading labeling."[47]

Dr. Robbins teaches that many vitamins that are **"natural"** never break down. They often contain additives, food allergens, sugar, artificial food coloring, flavoring, shellac, chlorine, and other potentially hazardous chemicals.

The word **"organic"** is also used commonly; implying something organically grown. Unfortunately the word "organic" means anything that contains a carbon atom which could mean a synthetic substance, not just organically-grown produce.

The word **"pure"** is legal because the product is the pure essence of the **chemical** molecule. The phrase **"vitamin complex"** is allowable because products could be from food sources, and contain **minute** quantities of the co-factors once in the food. The term **"from natural sources"** can refer to natural substances such as **corn sugar.** (For more information, see pages 69 and 70.)

I like what Dr. Robbins says about synthetic vitamins, "You don't **buy** synthetic vitamins—you **rent** them!" In other words, these toxic substances pass through the body unused at best and at worse, they cause harm to the kidneys.

How Can You Tell?

One way to check the solubility of a vitamin is to drop it in a glass of water and watch it break down. A natural, soluble vitamin will completely break away within 10-20 minutes. However, many drug store vitamins simply sit at the bottom of the glass, releasing colorings, dyes, or shellac.

Chemicals are toxic substances that need to be neutralized by the liver. **Our bodies are incredibly made, but that doesn't mean they have the ability to turn chemicals into nutrients.**

Another good way to tell if your vitamins are synthetic is to look at your urine. Synthetic vitamins, especially the B complex, make your urine yellow. Additionally, you can sometimes smell the odor of the vitamin in the urine. Don't waste your precious money on synthetic supplements which create expensive urine and may damage your health!

One of my female clients recently said, "I was really skeptical when you told me about your supplements. Every vitamin C I have ever tried upset my stomach and made me feel bad. I have never been able to take many vitamins. I would belch and get a stomachache. Except yours! I can even take your supplements on an empty stomach! And they don't turn my urine yellow."

Synthetic vitamin dealers would like you to believe that there's no difference between natural and synthetic, because their vitamins are cheaper to produce. But what good are they if they aren't even available to the body?

According to Dr. Royal Lee, vitamins that are isolated or synthesized in the laboratory are not natural, act as a drug, are toxic, and cause unbalance in the body chemistry. Natural vitamins are foods and they only work as nutrition when still contained in the whole complex, with all of the other synergists found in nature.[48]

I don't have room to print the testimonies of thousands of my clients who have been as surprised and delighted as I was with the results that they have received by taking **whole-food** supplements.

What's the Difference?

For you to really understand why synthetic and crystalline vitamins are a rip off, you need to understand how our government looks at supplements as compared to how the body uses food. While chemistry wasn't my favorite class, (I really preferred dance class!) I think it's vital to see the chemical composition of a vitamin to understand the difference between synthetics and whole-food supplements.

In each case, for every vitamin that has been discovered researchers identified one component and labeled it as the **organic nutrient.** In the mind of the FDA and most chemists or pharmacists, that is the entire vitamin.

For synthetic vitamin C the organic nutrient is ascorbic acid. **However, ascorbic acid is only a small percent of the natural C complex.** When you take the synthetic vitamin C, you never receive the other parts of the vitamin C complex, including bioflavonoids, tyrosinase, and P, K, and J factors.

For synthetic vitamin E the organic nutrient is alpha-tocopherol. But there are several other tocopherols, including beta-tocopherol, gamma-tocopherol, and delta-tocopherol, plus selenium and lipositols. Here's a recap of the vitamin C and E complexes as Dr. Royal Lee defined them:[49]

Vitamin C Complex	Vitamin E Complex
Ascorbic acid	Alpha-Tocopherol
Bioflavonoid Complex	Beta-Tocopherol
	Gamma-Tocopherol
Tyrosinase	Delta-Tocopherol
P, K, and J Factors	Lipositols
	Selenium

Similarly, beta carotene is only one of a number of carotenes including alpha, gamma and more. These never occur separately in foods, but only as a whole complex.[50]

I like to paraphrase Dr. Robbin's definition of this: **"To take the organic nutrient alone is like eating a banana peel without the banana and thinking that you ate the same nutrition as the banana!"**

He shows that there is a whole lot more in the food than just the organic nutrient. Look at the missing nutrients:

*Enzymes   *Precursors
*Co-enzymes   *Antioxidants
*Trace elements   *Activators

Additionally, there are numerous other naturally occurring synergistic micronutrients, some known and possibly others unknown. Any time you take synthetic or crystalline vitamins, you are missing **all** of this vital nutrition.

How To Read a Label

Let's look at the difference between synthetic and natural as it's shown on the labels. In both cases, the vitamin is listed on all supplements, e.g. vitamin A, but what is the source? Below is a comparison of the synthetic vitamin name(s) (or organic nutrient) and the whole-food natural source. On synthetic labels, **all** you'll see is the vitamin name. **On a natural label, you'll also see a list of known foods that contain the whole vitamin complexes.**

Vitamin	Synthetic Name	Natural Source
Vitamin A	Acetate, Palmintate, Retinol, Beta Carotene	Carrot powder Fish oils
Vitamin B1	Thiamine mononitrate Thiamine hydrochloride	Yeast Yeast
Vitamin B3	Niacin	Yeast
Vitamin B6	Pyridoxine hydrochloride	Yeast
Vitamin C	Ascorbic Acid	Rose hips Buckwheat juice
Vitamin E	D-alpha tocopherol or dl-alpha or d-alpha succinate	Wheat germ oil Peavine juice

Dr. Robbins further explains:

> The problem is that when the body is lacking in nutrition, it's not lacking in one isolated nutrient. Whatever the patient did to create the vitamin C deficiency, they at the same time, created a deficiency of **all** of the co-factors!

You can't get these from synthetic vitamins made in the laboratory that don't even have these co-factors. We don't have a synthetic vitamin deficiency; we have a food deficiency. Dr. Robbins says that there are at least 3,800 nutrient components in **one** food. To nourish the body and make up for nutrient deficiencies, **you have to give the body real food.** You can only get this by supplementing the body with whole-food supplements.

Why Bother To Eat?

I love science fiction movies and books. So often I notice scenarios where people just eat instant foods from some type of computer microwave, or just take processed food pills. But as a nutritionist, I can't help thinking what they don't show: The captain and crew are tired, constipated, and their hemorrhoids are acting up again!

If we really could get vitamins from vitamin pills which have been isolated and fractionated from the original food, then **why should we bother to eat real food at all? We can't.** We need whole-food nutrition from either the whole foods themselves (fresh fruits and vegetables, for example) which is best, or at least from dried whole-food supplements, not man-made chemical counterparts posing as food.

When I switched to whole-food natural supplements, my clients and I noticed a great difference. They reported feeling better within days. After the appropriate nutritional biochemical tests were nutritionally analyzed, I found that their health profiles improved consistently and dramatically. And their ability to lose weight naturally was greatly improved. We've even helped save many lives. I had one client tell me, "When I came to see you, I was planning to die; now I'm planning to live!"

We've been talking about vitamin supplements; let's take a moment to discuss minerals.

What About Minerals?

Both animals and people need minerals. Even microscopic organisms in the soil need trace minerals. But as

71

I said earlier, mineral-deficient soil has resulted in mineral deficient plants and people. So we need minerals, perhaps even more importantly than vitamins. There are so many different types of minerals. How do you know which to choose?

Here's more chemistry, but hang on; we'll get through it! Minerals in the earth are inorganic or dead. Our body can't use inorganic minerals because their molecular weight or size is too large to pass through the intestinal lining. We depend on plants to transform minerals from the soil into an organic form that we can use. This process is called **chelation**, which is the attachment of an amino acid to the mineral, making it usable by the body. The best way to get minerals is from whole foods that have been dried with a low temperature so none of the nutrition or enzymes are destroyed.

Let's take calcium for example. There are many different forms of calcium on the market. However, various forms of calcium not only have different absorption rates, but they also contain different amounts of actual calcium.

When most people need calcium, they look for a supplement with 1,000 or more milligrams on the label. However, few calcium supplements provide you with this amount.

According to nutritionist Doug Grant, calcium citrate is only 21% calcium. **He explains that if you eat 1,000 milligrams of calcium citrate, you are really only getting 210 milligrams of calcium.** In addition, less than 30% of the 210 milligrams of calcium is actually absorbed at the cellular level for use by the body.[51]

In other words, of the 210 milligrams of calcium contained, your body may only receive 60 to 70 milligrams. There's a huge difference! So don't be fooled by the "label milligram" game. (More about the milligram hype in synthetic vitamins in chapter 9.)

Are there any good mineral products on the market? It depends on how they are chelated. So the question is, "Which is the most efficient chelating agent?" According to Dr. Robbins, the softer agents are more efficient, for example, lactate, citrate, and gluconate.

Forms of minerals that aren't recommended include: Oxides, sulfates, chlorides, phosphates and hydroxides. Avoid harder chelating agents such as calcium carbonate (Tums, which is ground-up rocks) and oyster shell supplements. These forms are extremely hard for your body to assimilate.

And some forms are not only difficult to assimilate but they are harmful in the long run. (See chromium picolinate in chapter 8, page 79.)

How effectively a nutritional supplement is absorbed is far more important than how much is taken. Here's a good example of bad absorption.

Hugh St. Onge, a friend, sent me a report from the Nutrition Clinic in Chesterfield, Missouri. They have an x-ray of a woman, who had just delivered a baby, prior to life-saving surgery. It showed her intestinal tract blocked with some 90 pharmaceutical grade iron tablets that never passed through her intestinal wall!

Many clients ask me about liquid organic minerals. Many of these products contain more than 70 minerals. Here is a great example of thinking that if a little is good, more is better. We require just a trace of these precious minerals, and larger doses than are found naturally in food can upset our biochemistry. Taking too much zinc too long without balancing it with copper, for example, can upset the copper balance in your body. High levels of copper are linked to irritability, anger and rage. (No, not everything can be blamed on PMS!)

Besides, many people get plenty of minerals already, especially potassium, sodium and chloride. So additional quantities of these are often unnecessary. That's probably why there are no RDAs for these minerals.

And finally, the question is not whether the mineral is in the liquid or solid form, the question again goes back to how it was chelated. For example, you can find a liquid calcium carbonate, which is not as absorbable as a liquid calcium citrate or lactate.

Additionally, many of these formulas contain toxic minerals like aluminum and arsenic. So rather than looking for megadoses of minerals, try to get your minerals from whole foods or whole-food supplements.

Colloidal Minerals

Colloidal minerals have become quite popular, too. But I've never seen any scientific research that supports the use of colloidal minerals.

According to Dr. Robbins, the colloidal form of minerals can be absorbed because the molecule size is small. **But they are not chelated.** The chelation part is necessary for both absorption and utilization once the mineral is in the body.

As I said earlier, the best way to get minerals is through chelation, which means the minerals are bound or attached to an amino acid. If minerals are not absorbed in this way, they can become toxic. Few companies are willing to do this, since the process is more expensive.

Your stomach knows the difference. Chelated minerals from whole-food sources can be taken on an empty stomach without any problems. Now you know why you get a stomachache after taking colloidal minerals.

So how dangerous are these synthetics? You will understand more about synthetic vitamins in chapter 8.

Chapter Eight

Do Your Vitamins Help or Hurt You?

You've probably seen the television pharmaceutical commercials regarding such ailments as arthritis or high cholesterol. After they tell you all the benefits of the drug, they then list 10 or more side effects ranging from headaches to impotency. And it seems like almost everything causes diarrhea! Surprisingly, people still buy and take these drugs when there are often dietary and natural whole-food supplement solutions to most of these problems.

Perhaps you've read about the benefits of taking vitamin E, for example, to prevent strokes, so you went out and bought some. (You might have even taken it.) You assume that it will protect you from heart disease. But the idea of the vitamin hurting you is quite foreign, right?

When I was nearly 40 pounds overweight, I read hundreds of health books, and I bought lots of vitamins. These various authors had lots of rules; such as to take calcium at night, or take iron alone, and so on. Soon, taking my pills became a full-time job! I wondered, though, do these supplements interfere with each other? Can they be dangerous?

Author and nutritionist Dr. Vic Shayne gives an example of how vitamins can cause unbalance in our chemistry.

> An athlete may discover the need for zinc which he then supplements by the handful only to accidentally impair his supply of vitamin A, vitamin C, hormones, iron and copper. Copper deficiency, in turn, can increase blood cholesterol.[52]

Then the athlete goes to his doctor who gives him cholesterol-lowering medication all because he unknowingly threw off his mineral balance!

I've seen firsthand dozens of vitamins that don't work because my clients have brought me so many products that I now have a large file. They include "magical cures" that prevent aging that were loaded with sugar, and a weight-loss product that made them gain weight! Often these products come with a beautiful, full-color, 26-page magazine convincing you that you need this latest product. After they make their money, you never hear about it again. (The least they could do is use the same person in the "before and after" pictures!)

Why Vitamins Don't Always Work

In the last chapter, I said that synthetic supplements can and do create nutritional imbalances. Here's why. Scientists take things apart to see how they work. Once they identify which vitamin in a particular food affects a specific function, then they think that is the **only** part you need. They assume that the isolated nutrient works the same way when it's no longer a part of the whole-food complex. They don't.

A vitamin that is no longer in a food isn't natural and doesn't work like the food. Since they are a fractionated or isolated part, they work, but as a "drug-like" or pharmacological substance, not as a true nutrient. They may seem to work, but they are not feeding the cells with the nutrients needed by our chemistry to sustain life.

Nutraceuticals

The term "nutraceuticals" has become quite popular in nutritional flyers and advertisements. They sound health promoting, but are they?

Nutraceuticals are nutritional supplements that are isolated fractions of phytochemicals and whole foods. Here are a few examples. Beta carotene comes from carrots, alpha-tocopherol (vitamin E) comes from vegetable oils, and lycopene comes from tomatoes.

In an interview, Dr. Robbins explains,

> When we isolate a single component of food, thus taking it out of context for what the body is used to having, and then concentrate it as in a vitamin, it takes on a drug-like effect. For example, give a child an apple, and his behavior is fine; give him extracted sugar from the apple, and he becomes hyperactive.

We think of a nutraceutical as "natural," yet they are most often synthetic nutrients. As Dr. Bruce West writes,

> Even though synthetic beta carotene has been shown to make some cancers worse, it is being sold as a "nutrient." Beta carotene is just one of hundreds of carotenes which are just one of hundreds of nutrients found in fruits and vegetables. Do you think that isolating one factor among thousands and then making it synthetically makes sense?[53]

Dr. West says that the research so often used in advertisements to sell people on the benefits of these products always refers to the benefits that came from the **whole food,** while often selling you the **isolated or fragmented part.**

Food supplements made from whole specific plants and raw materials are rich in certain vitamins and phytochemicals. They need everything in perfect balance: Vitamins, minerals, trace elements, phytochemicals, and enzymes, so they work as whole food, not as a drug or stimulant.

Clinical Research

So what about the results from studies of isolated or fragmented vitamins? Here are a few journal references which validate the reason why synthetic vitamins are ineffective and can even be dangerous.

Vitamin A

This first example compares the test results of a synthetic vitamin to a real food source. It shows that the extract of beta carotene was not as effective as dried carrots in treating a skin disease.

> Stephenson found that a crude extract of dried carrot when added to a fat lacking in vitamin A conferred upon it growth promoting properties and protected rats from xerophthalmia while pure carotene extracted from carrots was without effect.[54]

Vitamin B

The study below was originally published in the *Journal of Nutrition* in 1939 by Dr. Barnet Sure. It warns us about the use of thiamine, a synthetic B1 vitamin and its link to sterility.

> (In rats) a daily dose of 100 (micrograms) of thiamin results in female sterility in the second generation. A daily dose of 200 (micrograms) of thiamin produces toxic effects in lactation in the third generation. A daily dose of 400 (micrograms) of thiamin results in entire failure in lactation in the third generation.[55]

The first group of rats became sterile after the first generation; the second and third groups couldn't feed their young. Even in humans, without proper nutrition, every generation gets weaker. That's why children can be born with what used to be adult diseases.

Synthetic vitamins are deficient because they do not contain the naturally-occurring nutritional counterparts from food that accompany the B vitamins and make them active in your body. These include trace minerals, enzymes, phytochemicals, and every other B vitamin.

Vitamin C

The following statement from a *British Journal of Chemistry and Physics* article showed that bleeding didn't stop with synthetic ascorbic acid but it did with fruit juice. Citrus fruits as natural sources of vitamin C contain something in addition to pure ascorbic acid.

> Three cases of hemorrhagic intestinal disease did not improve after daily intravenous injections of ascorbic acid, but were cured by lemon juice.[56]

78

Plain old lemon juice worked better; makes you want to drink some natural lemonade!

Another study from the University of Leicester, UK, showed that synthetic vitamin C can **cause** free radical damage; natural sources of vitamin C **prevent** it:

> The researchers found that at the 500 milligram level, (synthetic) vitamin C promoted genetic damage by free radicals to a part of the DNA, the adenine bases, that had not previously been measured in studies of the vitamin's oxidative properties.

> Unlike the vitamin C naturally present in foods like orange juice, vitamin C as a [synthetic] vitamin is not an antioxidant.[57]

Vitamin D

Synthetic vitamin D is called viosterol. Here is a study published in the *New York State Medical Journal:*

> Vitamin D factor in viosterol and cod liver oil are not identical. Ten times as many vitamin D units in viosterol do not give as much protection as plain cod liver oil.[58]

Chromium Picolinate

A University of Alabama researcher reported, "The popular dietary supplement chromium picolinate may damage DNA, possibly increasing the risk of cancer."[59]

Chromium picolinate is a synthetic form of chromium which doesn't appear to be as effective for sweet cravings as the natural form which is naturally extracted from yeast. The natural form has the glucose tolerance factor (GTF). I've helped hundreds of people control their sugar cravings with this natural form of chromium.

Vitamin E

Judith DeCava reports that when vitamin E is separated from its natural synergists, it loses up to 99% of its potency.[60]

This next study compared separated, synthetic vitamin E with wheat germ, a natural source of vitamin E.

In one test study, the vitamin E deficient laboratory animals fed tocopherols died sooner than the control animals that received no vitamin at all.[61]

Not eating any vitamin E is better than taking synthetic vitamin E! Our bodies need the **entire** E complex, including **all** of the tocopherols: Alpha, beta, gamma and delta, as well as lipositol, selenium and other nutrients to prevent disease.

An Incredible Story

Here's the Dr. Royal Lee story which has been passed on through the years. It's a great example of the power of natural whole-food supplements and the dangers of synthetics.

When Dr. Royal Lee introduced Catalyn in 1929 and began distributing it to doctors and patients, the response to the product was tremendous. Doctors and patients not only wanted more Catalyn, but they also wanted more products. Dr. Lee did not want to be in the supplement business; he was an engineer and an inventor.

He took his blossoming vitamin company to two drug companies, both of whom were also developing "vitamin" products. Dr. Lee offered to "give" them everything—the farms, the equipment and their patents, and the processing techniques. One company rejected the offer, the other decided to test Dr. Lee's Catalyn product against their own products first.

The company took three groups of lab animals and starved them nearly to death. One group was fed nothing, the second group was given Catalyn, and the third group was given the company's chemical vitamins.

In the first thirty days, all the animals in the first group died. The animals in the Catalyn group improved only 25%. The animals in the chemical vitamin group improved about 50%. In the next thirty days, the animals in the Catalyn group improved another 25%, while the animals in the chemical vitamin group improved to nearly 100%—almost fully recovered.

At the end of the next thirty days (90 days in all) the animals in the Catalyn group continued to improve, about another 25%, while the animals in the chemical vitamin group were dead!

When you give a living organism nutrients that are in an unnatural ratio to their bodies, it actually **causes imbalances** and deficiencies, leading eventually to disease and death.

The drug company was amazed. They decided to evaluate what it would cost to manufacture Dr. Lee's products—owning, operating, and maintaining the farms and the factory, and what their profits could be.

To make a large bottle of Catalyn, it takes 25 pounds of organic fruits and vegetables. In order for them to maintain their customary profit margin, they would have to sell Catalyn at $30 a bottle (in 1929 dollars). Because this was far too expensive, they rejected Dr. Lee's offer. Instead, Dr. Lee introduced Catalyn and his new company Standard Process, Inc., in 1929 at a cost of $6 a bottle.

More than 70 years later, it retails for only $9! I still think Catalyn is unfortunately one of the best kept secrets in the country. Standard Process is now sold only through healthcare professionals. It's my favorite whole-food supplement company and I've had most success with their products.

The majority of the thousands of clients I've counseled have improved their health dramatically by taking whole food supplements.

A client named Kim said, "I was very sick when I came to see Lorrie. Exhausted, I went to several doctors who all told me that 'it was all in my head.' I found Lorrie and now I am doing absolutely fantastic. Every symptom is gone."

After having her thyroid oblated through nuclear medicine (her doctors gave no other option for treating her diagnosed Grave's disease) my client Cathy was supposed to remain on thyroid replacement hormones for life.

She sought my help because she still struggled with fatigue, depression and weight gain. Her health profile pointed to chronic fatigue syndrome. Ten months later, with Standard Process supplements and modified eating habits, she no longer struggles with fatigue and depression. Her weight gain has stopped, and she is beginning to lose weight. And she's been completely medication free for seven months.

Supplements Compared to Drugs

The natural whole-food supplements that I am using in my practice are healthy and safe. Drugs, even when prescribed by physicians, are dangerous. Realize, too, that prescription and over-the-counter drugs kill between 100,000 and 200,000 people in the U.S. a year.

Recently, one of my clients went to her doctor about a rash. She read the label on a drug he had prescribed which said that after taking it, she could have kidney failure within a year! And people are concerned about taking our whole-food supplements! Go figure!

You might have read articles throughout the years stating that people who took vitamin E supplements **still** experienced heart attacks. Or people who took vitamin C **still** experienced hardening of the arteries. **All of these studies were done on synthetic vitamins, not whole-food supplements.**

Synthetic or man-made vitamins are toxic and may cause many adverse reactions, some as serious as sterility. But more importantly, synthetic or isolated vitamins never fix the original deficiency in the first place.

So let's look at the next issue of high-potency vitamins.

Chapter Nine

Potency: If a Little Is Good, Is More Better?

The other day, one of my clients stopped me as he was leaving my office and said, "Wait a minute!" This vitamin C that you just sold me only has 6 milligrams of vitamin C on the label. That's too low! I need lots of vitamin C to prevent disease!"

Like so many of my clients, I was taught that in order for vitamin C to be effective, we had to take large doses of it. After all, we were all looking for healthier alternatives to drug therapy, and vitamin therapy in large doses made sense.

But throughout the years, I noticed that not everyone got better with larger doses, and articles surfaced saying that larger doses could be dangerous. **How do you explain the apparent contradictions when it comes to dosing supplements?**

Many of my questions were answered when I understood the great difference between the source of the nutritional supplement, or natural whole-food supplements compared to synthetic vitamins.

Because most practitioners using supplements practice pharmacology rather than healing with whole-food nutrition, switching over to whole-food supplements can sometimes be confusing. Most commercial vitamins are based on pharmacology, or drug-like effects, rather than true nutrition. One of the most common problems is trying to figure out the number of milligrams of a particular vitamin in a whole-food supplement.

In his class, Dr. Robbins gives three myths we commonly hear about the potency of vitamins.

1. If a little is good, a lot must be better.

2. The higher the dosage, the faster the nutritional deficiency will be met.

3. Potency is determined by how high the milligram is.

None of these statements is true. But this is just another example of how misleading labels and popular nutritional information can be.

A Better Definition of Potency

The problem with this is, when studying synthetic or crystalline vitamins, a vitamin might appear to work at the beginning, but after the initial phase of metabolizing the vitamin, this process stops working. Why? Because your body has had to stop to search and then pull vitamins from its cells and tissues to make up for the missing nutritional pieces in the synthetic or crystalline, high-dose vitamins. So now you have a worse deficiency than before you started.

Potency or **effectiveness** is related to how "whole" the nutrient is, not how many milligrams it contains. As Judith DeCava aptly reports: **"A minute amount of a vitamin in its whole food form is more effective nutritionally than a large amount of a vitamin fraction."**[62]

Many times we are told that we need 1,000 milligrams of vitamin C. Any time we see high milligrams, it has to be an isolated fragment because natural substances don't have high milligrams. High-dose vitamin C, for example, contains ascorbic acid, but it's only one of six parts of the complete vitamin C. Furthermore, it was known over a half century ago that attempting to separate nutrients greatly decreases their strength.[63] Therefore these high milligram, isolated nutrients are less potent, not more potent.

It's easy to understand the idea of real potency when you consider what we've said about whole-food supplements. **We need the whole nutritional complex, not just high amounts of one organic nutrient to fix the deficiency.**

So potency isn't about how high the milligram level is, even though that's what we've always been taught. Potency is really about how complete the nutrition in the supplement is and how well it's delivered to the cells. This is known as "bioavailability."

For example, I commonly use a low-potency vitamin B called Cataplex B (between 5-20 mg.) which is far more effective than 50 or 100 mg. of synthetic B. Most of my clients are amazed at how much better they feel on the B that I recommend. Whole-food supplements don't give you an artificial burst of energy that quickly passes. Instead, they provide a constant, health-promoting energy source that lasts throughout the day.

Dr. Royal Lee said that **the whole food B complex is somewhere between 10 to 50 times more potent than a synthetic vitamin.**[64] For example, the label on the Standard Process Cataplex B supplement lists the Thiamine as .96 mg; Niacin as 20.44 mg. and B6 about .95 mg. While the whole complex isn't listed on the label, you can tell the entire B complex is present by the listed sources which are nutritional yeast and bovine liver powder, both of which contain the entire B complex. Dr. Lee also identified vitamin B4 as vital to our health. However, since there is no technology developed that can extract B4, all synthetic and crystalline vitamin B supplements lack B4 (except Standard Process or any whole herb that contains B vitamins). Taking synthetic and crystalline supplement forms eventually leads to serious vitamin B deficiencies.

We Can't Handle Them

Dr. Joel Robbins says it this way:

> The problem with taking partial nutrients as in isolated vitamins is that in order to use that food, **the body has to make up the difference with its own reserves.** Here's an example. There are more than 270 nutrients in an apple. The most you can extract from a multiple vitamin is about 50. If your body uses these 50, it has to complete the picture by supplying the remaining 220 nutrients.

We've identified many nutrients that nature provides. But there are hundreds of nutrients, if not more, that we haven't identified. We need them all. We attempt to provide only a small percentage of the nutrients that nature would have provided in the first place.

Man tries to reproduce what nature made, but how can he reach that perfect balance? As with the apple example, how can you replace what you haven't even identified? Each food has every nutrient combined perfectly; it's the imbalance that causes deficiencies. **So by taking isolated synthetics, we run the risk of creating other imbalances or deficiencies.**

Our bodies are designed to use a balance of nutrients. Anything beyond that becomes toxic. Let's take the example of an orange which contains about 50 milligrams of vitamin C. Most supplements contain far more than that—1,000 milligrams. To get that amount in food, you would have to eat more than 20 oranges. How many oranges could you eat? We could eat between 3 to 5 oranges in one sitting. That means between 150-250 milligrams of vitamin C. Any extra vitamin C is considered an overload to the body. No wonder people get diarrhea from taking so much vitamin C.

Taking large amounts of these vitamins causes an increased metabolism; they act as a stimulant, not a healing agent. At one level, they may fulfill a vitamin or mineral deficiency. However, they are providing symptomatic relief by stimulating the body. **Nutrients in excess become toxic to the body.** So the body has to re-prioritize from healing to eliminating the concentrated inorganic vitamins.

Here's a good example of the difference between synthetics and natural supplements. Most of the time, people feel better taking supplements. But if you ask them if they have been able to reduce the amount of supplements they take, they usually say that they have to increase. They need to take **more** to feel as good as they did when they started with them. In my practice, when we take care of the deficiency, we can begin to eliminate the supplements as their diet becomes sufficient.

What about the toxic side effects? There is a cost to eliminating these supplements through the urine. If the vitamins have a non-nutritive coating, or sugar, or food colorings, these all have to be neutralized in the liver before they are excreted. Why keep putting in toxic material?

I was trained to keep increasing my dose of vitamin C until I got diarrhea—then slowly start backing down until it stops; that's when you know you have the right dose. But what really happens is that large amounts of synthetic vitamin C are **toxic,** so your body has to eliminate it, which causes the diarrhea.

Ask a Different Question

We need a new perspective regarding whole-food supplements. Whole-food supplements come from whole foods. We are not using them to inject a zillion milligrams of a certain nutrient into the body for a drug-like effect. We use them for the food complexes that are missing in today's devitalized diets. We are trying to bring balance to the body.

So instead of asking does a vitamin have so many milligrams, we should ask: "Does it contain the entire combination of nutrients just like it's found in natural foods such as carrots or beets?"

Our bodies need **all** of the co-factors (see page 66) to make a vitamin work. So your body doesn't need high amounts; it only needs the whole complex.

Most vitamin/mineral supplements on the market are refined or only part of a food. We weren't designed to eat partial foods. We're designed to eat real foods which come with a full range of nutrients.

We Need Whole Foods

Natural fruits and vegetables don't have high quantities of nutrients. As Dr. Robbins said earlier, nature made it quite difficult to eat enough oranges to overdose on the vitamin C complex. However, when we take large quantities of concentrated synthetic vitamins, the body has to work overtime to keep the excesses from disrupting its delicate chemistry.

The Dangers of High Potency

Earlier we gave the dangers of synthetic vitamins; now let's look at the dangers of excess. So often we have this "if a little is good, even more is better" mentality about vitamin supplements.

Think about your diet. Will you be healthier by taking in double, triple, or even higher amounts of your carbohydrates, fats, and proteins? No.

Most high-potency vitamin B pills are thiamine. Your body can only absorb 2-5 mgs. daily, yet most B vitamins contain 50 to 100 mg.

According to an article by Dr. Royal Lee in "The Fallacy of High Potency in Vitamin Dosage," too much of a vitamin causes the reverse effect:

> But there is another principle that is little known, and highly important to this question of dosage. It is the fact that many vitamins may cause, in excess quantities, the same symptoms as are caused by their deficiency.
>
> Vitamin B1 in small doses can cure herpes zoster; large doses can cause herpes zoster.
>
> A deficiency in vitamin B1 causes symptoms similar to hyperthyroidism. An excess of the same vitamin causes similar symptoms.[65]

More Examples

We have been misled into thinking that massive doses (called megadoses) of vitamins are beneficial.

In his article called "America's Very Dangerous Vitamin Craze," Dr. Victor Herbert, Professor of Medicine at Mount Sinai School of Medicine says: "In amounts far in excess of the Reference Daily Intake (RDI), vitamins become drugs—with toxic side effects."[66] His recommendation is only 30 I.U. of vitamin E.

Whole-food supplements, since they are made from whole foods, are naturally low-dose and therefore effective and safe in any amount.

Contradictory Reports

You probably have read that vitamin E is vital for fertility. Look at this research published in the *Medical Tribune:*

It has been shown that antioxidants vitamin C and vitamin E, when taken in frequent megadose amounts, depress sperm motility, and therefore, decrease fertility.[67]

Perhaps you've even heard contradictory reports on the benefits of antioxidants.

Megadoses of vitamin C blunt the beneficial effects of chemotherapy treatment for breast cancer. Cancer cells have numerous receptors for vitamin C, making the vitamin C act as a growth tonic for cancer cells.[68]

Millions of people take high doses of antioxidants every day, but they are still sick and getting sicker. Any time high or megadoses are being used, they are using synthetic vitamins, because whole-food supplements are naturally low dose. These studies are referring to the damaging effect of using isolated, synthetic ascorbic acid in high doses.

Megadoses of Vitamin D

Dr. Royal Lee cited one report in the *Journal of the American Medical Association* where children were poisoned by the recommended doses for the prevention of rickets. He also wrote:

> Vitamin D in overdose reverses the effect of mild dosage. In a deficiency, there is a negative calcium balance; in excess, there is also a negative calcium balance. Only the nutritional dosage promotes assimilation of calcium.[69]

The Bottom Line

Milligram quantity is not nearly as important as the presence of all the organically combined synergists. Potency is not determined by quantity.

> Dr. Agnes Fay Morgan a nutritional authority, performed a laboratory experiment with so-called 'high-potency' vitamins, the synthetic fractions which are used to 'enrich' foods such as refined 'white' flour. The laboratory animals on the 'high-potency enriched diet' did not live as long as those on the same low vitamin diet without the enrichment.[70]

Dr. Morgan said that animals fed on the synthetic vitamin enriched diet died long before the other animals. Why? Because high-potency vitamins aren't food so they act like a drug or stimulant, not as a healing agent. On the contrary, whole-food supplements help the body to repair.

It's impossible to compare doses for a synthetic vitamin with doses of a whole-food supplement because they are two different substances. One is an isolated synthetic substance, the other is a food complex.

I have been using whole-food supplements for several years, and my clients who are used to taking higher dosages are amazed at how well natural supplements work.

So let's wind this up by looking at what you really need.

Chapter Ten

What Do You Really Need?

One of the most common questions I am asked is: "Can I get all of my nutrition from food? Why do I have to take supplements?" And usually this is the person who has reserved parking at Krispy Kreme doughnuts!

My reply is, "Yes, if you grow your own food on a farm where you practice organic gardening, eat animals that grazed on grass, fish in uncontaminated waters, reduce your stress, don't eat fast food or junk food, and drink pure water—no problem!"

When a client comes to see me, the first thing I do is discover what their goals are—why they came to see me. After I finish the consultation, and we talk about supplements, I like to tell my clients what supplements can and can't do. What they can do is help make up nutritional deficiencies and bridge the gap of deficient foods and soil.

What they can't do is as important.

What Whole-Food Supplements Can't Do

1. **They can't replace a good, balanced diet** and regular meals. Green vegetables, both raw and cooked are vital for good health along with protein, fruit, and unprocessed carbohydrates.

2. **They can't replace regular exercise.** You don't have to lift weights, but try to get more movement in your daily life. (Not just sliding back and forth to mix the hot and cold water in the bath tub!) Exercise increases the great benefits of whole-food supplementation.

3. **They can't replace a good attitude.** We live in a world with a "quick fix" mentality. People are quick to take a drug to handle difficult times. While I agree with consulting your doctor, I would also check for folic acid, B12, and iron deficiencies, or hormone imbalances. St. John's Wort and other herbs are helpful, too. However, in addition to taking supplements and making dietary changes, I encourage people to see a counselor to help them think on the positive side of things. (For more help in this area, see my book, *Why Can't I Stay Motivated?*)

Getting Started

When I first interview a client, I identify the most important 3-5 nutrients they need. Many times, they are low in a dozen or so nutrients, but I usually only start with a few. For one thing, I like to "put out fires" by addressing their immediate concerns. Secondly, I try to be sensitive to how many supplements they can take, as well as their pocketbook. By their follow-up appointment, they have a good idea of how they like the supplements. Because I use whole-food supplements, I'm surprised if people **don't** feel better.

To help them make these important changes in their diet and begin taking whole-food supplements, I give every client a daily dosage sheet, a free pill box and a suggested meal plan. (For more help in designing your life around good nutrition, see my book, *Why Can't I Stay Motivated?*) Let's look now at how to start a vitamin/mineral program.

What Should We Take?

Your body is not like your car—there is no gauge to show you that something is wrong. No computer chip to say, "You're low in iron. You need more magnesium." And let's face it. It's much easier to get replacement parts for your car than it is for your body! So how do you know what you need?

I'll give you some recommendations that would benefit most people. Your "natural" healthcare professional (See page 100) may have additional recommendations, based on blood tests, symptom surveys, a hair analysis, urine or saliva tests, nutritional tests, or other types of testing.

Take your supplements as directed on the bottle or as directed by your natural healthcare professional. Nutritional healing takes time. I encourage my clients to allow a minimum of 3-6 months (or even years) because we're dealing with the **cause** of the problem (multiple deficiencies), not just the symptoms.

Be careful where you get your advice, though. If you see a copy of *Nutrition for Dummies* in their office, or your nutritionist thinks that anemia is a country near Russia, I would find someone else!

Take Whole-Food Supplements

Throughout this book, I've stressed the importance of taking whole-food supplements. Dr. Royal Lee, the original developer of the whole-foods supplement company, Standard Process, was a graduate dentist, an electronic engineer and innovator, a physiological researcher and a manufacturing biochemist. He held over 50 patents at the time of his death.

Many people believe that Royal Lee was a nutritional genius, years ahead of his time. He believed that only nutrients kept within their natural and concentrated form could effectively fill any nutritional gap. Since I'm most familiar with Standard Process, I'll use them as examples.

1. A Whole-Foods Multiple Vitamin/Mineral: My preference is Catalyn which is head and shoulders above any other multiple on the market. Many clients ask me about their "one-a-day" vitamins. In order to explain the difference, we have to compare what's on the labels. **Most synthetic "one-a-day" vitamins contain one part—the organic nutrient—of each complex.** For example, one client showed me his $30 synthetic vitamin. For vitamin C, it lists "ascorbic acid," for vitamin E, it lists "alpha-tocopherol," and so on. Its label indicates that it only contains cheap, chemical versions of each organic nutrient.

Catalyn, which retails for $9 (at the time of this writing), contains **each entire complex.** Compared to the typical one-a-day, Catalyn contains hundreds of thousands of nutrients from many whole-food sources. For example, rather than just thiamine, it contains the entire B complex which includes all of the B vitamins. Rather than just alpha-tocopherol, it contains the entire E complex including alpha, beta, gamma, and delta tocopherols, as well as selenium, xanthine, lipositols, and much more. Rather than just ascorbic acid, it contains the bioflavonoids, tyrosinase, and P, K and J factors, and so on. Unfortunately, there's not enough room to list all of these nutrients on the label.

Additionally, Catalyn works as a catalyst for hundreds of chemical reactions in the body, optimizing the benefits provided by the supplements.

Dr. Lee wrote as far back as 1938 that there are many parts of the complex, and even many versions of each complex. (Hope this isn't getting too complex!)

> In our slight present knowledge of vitamin chemistry, we have so far found four forms of vitamin A, six forms of vitamin B, three forms of vitamin C, twelve forms of vitamin D, etc.
>
> Ascorbic acid (the main ingredient in most multiple vitamins) has proven quite useless in controlling a condition of bleeding gums, loose teeth and black and blue spots (pseudo bruises) that indicate a definite scurvy condition. [71]

Avid label readers looking for maximum amounts of certain nutrients won't find them on the Catalyn label. As with all whole-food supplements, Catalyn is packed with **every nutrient complex** from organic sources. They are the vitamins, minerals, and trace elements normally found in a multiple vitamin.

Catalyn is so comprehensive, I use it (or Cyrofood which contains more fiber) as part of my pre-natal protocol. For example, when Michelle came to see me, she had been on her pre-natal for four months. She reported, "When I switched to Catalyn, within two weeks I was feeling much better!" I've seen great results using Catalyn compared to synthetic, pre-natal vitamins on the market. Women reported feeling better, having more energy, and their pregnancies were much easier.

2. A Digestive Enzyme: I use Zypan, Multizyme, Zymex, Okra-Pepsin or Gastrex, depending on the condition. (Your natural health professional who gave you this book will help you decide which one is appropriate.)

3. An Essential Oil Supplement: This contains essential fatty acids important in making prostaglandins for proper hormone function. **Linum B6** is the Standard Process flaxseed oil supplement.

In addition to these, here are additional supplements that might be appropriate.

4. A Vitamin B Complex: Many people who are overweight, fatigued or exhausted are deficient in the B complex vitamins so vital for proper carbohydrate metabolism. **Cataplex B** is one of the best B complex supplements that I have ever used which contains the entire B complex. **The label lists doses between 5-20 milligrams which are far more effective than the common 50 or 100 milligrams listed on synthetic B vitamin labels.**

5. An Antioxidant: If you are concerned about cancer, live in a polluted environment, or want a stronger preventive health program, take natural vitamins A, C, E and the mineral selenium which are antioxidants. There are several ways to get this protection from whole foods. Standard Process **Cataplex AC, ACP** or **OPC** with **Cataplex E** are great.

Remember, there is a big difference between what's on the label and what's inside. If you look at Cataplex E, for example, you'll see **5 I.U. of the entire E complex, which is far superior to 400-600 I.U. of just alpha-tocopherol.** The same goes for each of the supplements. A good rule of thumb is to follow the directions on the label, unless your natural healthcare professional has given you different instructions.

6. A Calcium/Magnesium Supplement or other bone building formula. It's especially good if you don't eat dairy products, and drink caffeinated beverages. I use **Calcium Lactate**, which is a vegetable-based calcium, with a proper ratio of calcium to magnesium. Magnesium deficiencies are even more common. I recommend **Magnesium Lactate.**

7. A Green Food Supplement: So many people don't eat the most protective foods: fresh fruits and vegetables. For those people, **SP Green Food** is great. It contains brussels sprouts, kale, alfalfa, and barley grass, all organically grown.

8. Probiotics or an Acidophilus Supplement is vital if you have yeast infections or use antibiotics frequently. **Lactenz** or **Zymex** or a combination of both are great.

In addition to the above list, your natural healthcare professional may recommend a particular "protocol" to help the body regain health. For example, I use Cataplex B, Multizyme, and Cataplex GTF or Diaplex to help people with sugar cravings and blood-sugar problems.

How Do You Take Them?

I encourage you to try to take your supplements three times a day with meals. If you can't take them with meals, then take them before or after you eat. If you can't manage to take them three times, then cut the dosage in half and take them twice a day. Just get them in every day!

Whole-food supplements, since they are food, nourish your body every time you take them. Some protocols call for 3 a day, and others 6 a day. Follow these recommendations; otherwise you won't get results, or you'll need the product longer. For example, if you only take 3 Cataplex GTF a day, it's not as effective for stopping sugar cravings as 6 a day. Until you get the right dose, you will keep needing the supplement.

What About "New and Improved" Products?

Every day I hear about "new" miracle cures, or "new" nutritional products. Frequently, my clients call, fax, or e-mail me about these products, which after investigation, are just a new synthetic or fractionated version of something that was there all along—real, whole foods.

Two popular examples are MSM and Co-Q10, which when isolated are synthetic. Most of these can be cheaply manufactured and sold at huge profits. Standard Process contains the whole-food versions of most of these "new" products. For example, Spanish Black Radish is a natural source of MSM. Cardio Plus is a natural source of Co-Q10, and so on.

Isolated amino acids are another example. So many young athletes are now taking isolated creatine; yet no one has done any long-term studies on their effects.

In every case, you are only getting parts of these sources, and your body has to complete the nutritional picture, causing nutritional deficiencies. According to Dr. Robbins, in the long-term, you don't win. In the short-term, you never solve the real problem.

Detoxification

Having helped so many clients with weight loss, I believe that some people won't ever be well until they detox their bodies. Having helped dozens of clients with this cleanse for the past 8 months, I can highly recommend the Standard Process Purification Program. There are three parts to this cleanse.

SP Cleanse: The different nutrients found in SP Cleanse can help the body cleanse by addressing both phase 1 and phase 2 parts of the liver detoxification process, promoting healthy liver functions.

SP Complete: A great nutritional powder that can be mixed with water to create a shake that provides essential vitamins and minerals as a daily protein supplement.

Gastro Fiber: This product contains whole-food and botanical ingredients plus their synergistic co-factors to provide natural, fiber-based, dietary support.

Nutrition for Your Pets, Too

Recently one of my clients sent me a label from their dog food. The ingredients included brown rice, barley, rice bran oil, fish meal, and the vital Omega 3 fatty acids. It's finally happened—dogs can now eat better than people! What's next? "One-a-day's" for your fish?

We already know that pets (such as Thumper, Buffy and Sofie, my assistant, Carolyn's pets) love Standard Process Products. For example, one client called telling us that her dog ate an entire bottle of Drenamin. Happily, dog and owner were fine! (But we encourage you to keep your supplements away from your pets and let them take their own!)

Standard Process has veterinary products to specifically address the needs of dogs and cats. Appropriately named Canine formulas for your dog, and Feline for your cat. (Sorry, no fish, gerbil or bird food available yet!)

Are Supplements Expensive?

According to Robert Crayhon, "Some say supplements are a waste of money. Americans spend more money on potato chips than they do on vitamins. Potato chips are packed with trans fats that cause free radical damage. The soda industry dwarfs the vitamin industry."[72]

I've heard people say, "Oh, those vitamin people. Always trying to get your money." But you never hear them say, "Oh, those soda people. Always trying to get your money!" Soda is junk; it does nothing for you—except rob you of vital nutrients which the vitamin supplements help you replace.

A Great Investment

When people first change their diets, adding more expense on top of a grocery-food budget can seem overwhelming. That's why I help people go through their diets and ditch all of the junk and nutrient-depleting foods. Instead of spending money on coffee and a donut in the morning, why not use that money to have a protein drink? As a bonus, you'll feel better, have more energy, and look better when you eat wholesome foods.

It costs money to stay healthy! There is no way around it. It is not cheaper to eat better or healthier. Yes, you may want to go and sell the family silver—it's still worth it.

You have to think of this as an investment in your health. Isn't it cheaper to spend money today and prevent heart disease than end up with a triple by-pass surgery operation 10 years later? This surgery costs upwards of $15-20 thousand dollars and could have been prevented! Which was the better investment?

Realize that the drug manufacturers dwarf the vitamin supplement industry, which grosses about 6 billion dollars a year. A single drug can gross sales between 5-10 billion dollars a year. There is a great difference between a $9 multiple vitamin and a $150 drug!

You Can Afford It

People are so funny. Often they tell me, "Oh, I'm so glad that I found you! You are an answer to my prayer!" A month later, however, these same people say, "I'm so sick of taking these vitamins! Do you realize how much money I've spent?" Never mind that they no longer have headaches, they can finally sleep through the night, they no longer crave sugar, and they have lost 20 pounds! And no longer are they spending any money on medications.

Do they ever say to their spouse, "I suppose we have to spend money on food this month!" No. We know that we need food. But we need supplements, too. Disease doesn't just reverse itself. We have to change our diets, and we all have to make up the nutritional deficiencies sooner or later.

People buy supplements every day and just take the manufacturer's word about how they are made and what's in them. They don't consider what type of supplement it is, or the integrity of the company selling them. Don't be tempted by cheap bargains that in the long run, only waste your money. Look for tried-and-true companies that have been on the market for a long time, such as the 70-year old Standard Process company. My practice has grown simply by word-of-mouth because of the great results we see year after year.

I'm results-oriented, and I am passionate about helping my clients get healthy. I can't afford **not** to have the best. I've mentioned Standard Process in this book. Standard Process (sold only through health professionals) is involved in every step of production. Each year, they rotate the crops they grow and change the acreage for each crop. Not only do they have the highest standard of professional supplements, but they have the best prices.

I can also recommend another product I use called Medi-Herb, which is a whole-food herbal company that shares the same philosophy as Standard Process. Whatever you buy, I encourage you to find whole-food supplements from a company that you can trust.

What Is a "Natural" Healthcare Professional?

The type of "natural" health professional you want to assist you in internal body detoxification and health improvement are Naturopathic Doctors (N.D.), Clinical Nutritionists (C.N.), Certified Clinical Nutritionists (C.C.N.), and any doctor (D.C., M.D., D.D., D.O., D.D.S., Ph.D.) or pharmacists who has studied and even completed post-graduate studies in Clinical Nutrition.

(For more information on Standard Process, talk to the professional who gave you this book or call 1-800-848-5061 to find a natural healthcare professional in your area.)

My prayers for great health are with you.

Food Sources of Vitamins

Vitamin A (animal sources)

Milk, egg yolks, cheese, beef liver, fatty fish (salmon), yogurt.

Beta Carotene (Pro vitamin A: vegetarian sources)

Carrots, sweet potatoes, spinach, corn, squash, peaches, collard greens, kale, sweet red peppers, tomatoes, watermelon, butternut squash, asparagus, beet greens, cantaloupe, broccoli, alfalfa.

Vitamin B1 (Thiamine)

Unrefined whole grain cereals, wheat germ, wheat germ oil, brewer's yeast, brazil nuts, sunflower seeds, egg yolks, oatmeal, milk, peanuts, green peas.

Vitamin B2 (Riboflavin)

Brewer's yeast, milk, yogurt, eggs, cheese, almonds, organ meats like beef liver, some leafy green vegetables and fish.

Vitamin B3 (Niacin)

Beef liver, red meat, fish, green vegetables, brewer's yeast, tofu, cereals, soybeans, wheat germ, wheat germ oil, chicken, rice polishings, eggs, peanuts, avocados, sesame seeds, cheese.

Vitamin B5 (Pantothenic Acid)

Brewer's yeast, whole grains, meat, avocado, salmon, organ meats, egg yolks, peanuts, muscle meats, royal jelly, chicken, crude molasses, milk.

Vitamin B6 (Pyridoxine)

Brewer's yeast, wheat bran and wheat germ, avocados, bananas, organ meats, soybeans, eggs, fish, poultry, meat, oats, peanuts, brown rice.

Vitamin B9 (Folic Acid)

Beef liver, organ meats, spinach, Brewer's yeast, rice bran, leafy greens, beets, carrots, liver, tuna fish, salmon, eggs, whole grains.

Vitamin B10 (PABA or Para-aminobenzoic Acid)

Brewer's yeast, whole grains, peanuts, wheat germ, molasses, eggs, soybeans.

Vitamin B12 (Cyancobalamin)

Sardines, beef, eggs, corn, salmon, tuna, milk, cheese, natural tamari (Japanese soy sauce).

Biotin

Egg yolks, sardines, brewer's yeast, beef liver, nuts, whole grain cereals, brown rice, mushrooms.

Vitamin C (Ascorbic Acid)

Citrus fruits, berries, melons, green leafy vegetables, tomatoes, red peppers, rose hips, broccoli, brussels sprouts, papaya.

Vitamin D

Natural sunlight, meat, fish and fish oils, (cod and halibut liver oil), sardines and herring, egg yolks, milk (fortified with D), butter.

Vitamin E

Wheat germ and wheat germ oil, other unrefined expeller pressed vegetable or seed oils, avocado, whole wheat, soy, green leafy vegetables, spinach, eggs, whole-grain cereals, almonds, hazelnuts, sunflower seeds.

Calcium

Milk, cheese, cottage cheese, yogurt, beef liver, green leafy vegetables, soybeans, wheat germ, tofu, sesame seeds, almonds, dried beans, broccoli.

Chromium

Brewer's yeast, liver, whole grains, bran, rice polishings, eggs, apples, blackstrap molasses, red meat.

Copper

Almonds, walnuts, molasses, black olives, vegetables, soybeans, liver, wheat germ, red meat and mushrooms.

Iodine

All seafood, sea vegetables, iodized sea salt, spinach, onions, prunes.

Iron

Blackstrap molasses, almonds, liver, egg yolks, fish, soybeans, nuts, avocados, parsley, prunes, raisins, spinach.

Magnesium

Wheat germ, whole-wheat bread, nuts, almonds, sesame seeds, figs, dark green vegetables, bananas, red meat, seafood, poultry.

Manganese

Rice polishings, brown rice, nuts, navy beans, red meat, green leafy vegetables, egg yolks, blackstrap molasses.

Phosphorus

Meat, cheese, egg yolks, fish, poultry, brewer's yeast, whole grains, almonds, wheat germ, rice polishings, sunflower seeds.

Potassium

Citrus fruits, apples, oranges, bananas, melons, grapes, cantaloupe, green leafy vegetables, mint leaves, blackstrap molasses, potatoes, sunflower seeds, raisins, figs, avocados, peanuts, dates.

Selenium

Seafood, wheat germ, whole grains, brazil nuts, brewer's yeast, onions, broccoli, garlic, eggs.

Silicon

Whole-grain cereals, fruits (skin), horsetail, soybeans, alfalfa sprouts, onions, nuts and seeds.

Sodium

Sea salt, milk, cheese, meat, seafood, celery.

Zinc

Oysters, liver, sunflower seeds, brewer's yeast, cheese, mushrooms, turkey, almonds, pumpkin seeds.

Protein

Complete proteins provide the eight necessary amino acids and are found in animal foods: Meat, eggs, milk, cottage cheese, yogurt, fish, and cheese. Incomplete proteins lack some essential amino acids and need to be combined with complimentary protein or animal proteins: For example, whole grains and beans.

Essential Fatty Acids

Omega 3 fatty acids are found in cold-water fish such as salmon, mackerel, sardines, cod, and tuna. The best plant sources of Omega 3 are flaxseeds, flaxseed oil and walnuts. Omega 6 fatty acids are found in sesame, safflower, corn and olive oils.

Soluble fibers

Pectin: Apples, beets, bananas, cabbage, citrus fruits, peas, okra, squash.

Mucilages and gums: Oats, beans, black beans, fennel seeds, flax seeds, garbanzo beans, guar gum, glucomman, kidney beans, lima beans, oat bran, pinto beans, psyllium seeds, red beans.

Insoluble fibers

Cellulose: Apples, bran, peas, green beans, lima beans, cabbage, carrots, whole grains, wheat flour, brussels sprouts.

Hemicellulose: Brussels sprouts, broccoli, bananas, beets, corn, pears, peppers.

Lignin: Grains, whole grain cereals, eggplant, green beans, strawberries, pears, radishes, tomatoes, cabbage, peaches.

Endnotes

1. World Health Organization Statistical Information (Web address: www.who.int/home-page)

2. National Center for Health Statistics, 2000 "Leading Causes of Death" (Web address: www.cdc.gov/nchs/fastats/lcod.htm.)

3. Patrick Quillin, Ph.D., *Beating Cancer With Nutrition* (Tulsa, OK: The Nutrition Times Press, Inc., 2001), p. 23.

4. World Health Organization (web address above)

5. Earl Mindell, *Prescription Alternatives* (Keats Publishing: Los Angeles, CA) 1998, p. 285.

6. Nathaniel Altman, "Nutrition and Watergate," *Health Quarterly,* April 1980, p. 72.

7. "Dietary Goals of the United States Select Committee on Nutrition & Human Needs," (Feb. 1977); United States Government Printing Office, Washington, D.C., p. 13.

8. Miles T. Bader, Dr., *4001 Food Facts and Chef's Secrets* (San Diego, CA: Mylin Enterprises, 1992), p. 241.

9. Shari Lieberman, Ph.D., *The Real Vitamin and Mineral Book* (Garden City Park, NY: Avery Publishers, 1997), p. 27.

10. Reprinted with permission from *Staying Healthy With Nutrition* by Elson Haas, M.D. Copyright 1992 by Elson Haas, M.D. Celestial Arts, Berkeley, CA. (Available from your local bookseller, by calling 800-841-2665, or by visiting www.tenspeed.com.), p. 430.

11. Dr. Don Colbert, *What You Don't Know May Be Killing You* (Lake Mary, FL: Siloam Press, 2000), p. 151.

12. Mark Virkler, *Eden's Health Plan: Go Natural* (Destiny Image Publishers, Shippensburg, PA), 1994, p. 70.

13. Patrick Quillin, Ph.D., *Beating Cancer With Nutrition* (Tulsa, OK: The Nutrition Times Press, Inc., 2001), pp. 71-72.

14. Lisa Messinger, *Why Should I Eat Better?* (Garden City Park, NY: Avery Publishers), 1993, p. 1.

15. Mark Anderson and Dr. Bernard Jensen, *Empty Harvest* (Garden City Park, NY: Avery Publishers), 1990, p. 1.

16. Mary June Parks, *Menu and the Mind* (Frankfort, KY: Parks Publishers, 1986), pp. 65-68.

17. Mary June Parks, p. 65, 71.

18. Dr. Royal Lee, "The Special Nutritional Qualities of Natural Foods," 1942, Report No. 4, pp. 38-39.

19. Dr. Royal Lee, p. 43.

20. Dr. Royal Lee, p. 41.

21. Dr. Royal Lee, p. 49.

22. Dr. Royal Lee, p. 34.

23. Dr. Royal Lee, p. 46.

24. Dr. Royal Lee, p. 48.

25. Ibid.

26. Brian Peskin, *Beyond the Zone* (Houston, TX: Noble Publishing, 1999), p. 11.

27. Lorrie Medford, *Why Can't I Lose Weight?* (Tulsa, OK: LDN Publishing, 1999), p. 143.

28. Brian Peskin, p. 121.

29. Vitamin News for October 1999: *Journal of the American Medical Association.*

30. *Life Extension*, "Nutritional Values Decline," March 2001, pp. 28-30.

31. Ibid, p, 29.

32. Reprinted with permission from *Staying Healthy Shopper's Guide* by Elson Haas, M.D. Copyright 1999 by Elson Haas, M.D. Celestial Arts, Berkeley, CA. (Available from your local bookseller, by calling 800-841-2665, or by visiting www.tenspeed.com.), p. 109.

33. Sue Frederick, *How to Shop A Natural Foods Store* (Boulder, CO: New Hope Communications, 1994), p. 38.

34. Ibid, p. 38.

35. Elson Haas, M.D., p, 111.

36. Ibid.

37. Elson Haas, p. 105.

38. Sue Frederick, p. 38, 39.

39. Ibid.

40. Max Gerson, *A Cancer Therapy* (Bonita, CA: The Gerson Institute, 1990), p. 14.

41. *Journal of National Cancer Institute,* Vol. 84, July 1992, p. 997.

42. Reprinted with permission from Judith DeCava, M.S., LNC, *The Real Truth About Vitamins and Antioxidants* (West Harmouth, MA: A Printery, 1997), p. 42.

43. Judith DeCava, M.S., LNC, p. 38.

44. Judith DeCava, M.S., LNC, p. 117, 121.

45. Gilbert Levin, Ph. D. "Discussing Optical Isomers or Asymmetrical Molecules with Atomic Arrangements That Are Mirror Images of Each Other," *Discover,* 1981.

46. Dr. Royal Lee, "How and Why Synthetic Poisons Are Being Sold as Imitations of Natural Foods and Drugs," December 1948.

47. "Vitamin E: Biochemistry and Health Implications," Vol. 570, *Annals of the NY Academy of Sciences:* NY, 1989.

48. Dr. Royal Lee, "How and Why Synthetic Poisons Are Being Sold as Imitations of Natural Foods and Drugs," December 1948.

49. Judith DeCava, M.S., LNC, p. 212, 214.

50. Judith DeCava, M.S., LNC, p. 65.

51. Doug Grant *The Cutting Edge* (Mesa, AZ: Optimal Health Systems, Spring 2000), p. 1.

52. Vic Shayne, Ph.D. *Whole Food Nutrition* (Lincoln, NE: iUniverse.com, Inc., 2000), p. 2.

53. Bruce West, *Health Alert,* Vol. 17, Issue 7., p. 8.

54. Sherman, H., and Smith, S., *The Vitamins,* Second Edition (NY: The Chemical Catalog Company, Inc., NY, 1931), p. 244.

55. Sure, B., *Journal of Nutrition,* Vol. 18:2, pp. 187-194, August 10, 1939.

56.   Lund, H., and Elmby, A., *Abstract from British Journal of Chemistry and Physics,* August 1938, pg. 678.

57.   "High Doses of Vitamin C May Be Harmful," Leicester, UK, *Nature* 392:559, April 9, 1998.

58.   De Sanctis, A., and Craig, J., *New York State Journal of Medicine* 34, 16:712-714, 1934.

59.   March 24, 1999 New York (Reuters) a University of Alabama researcher reported at the American Chemical Society's annual meeting in Anaheim, CA.

60.   Judith DeCava, M.S., LNC, p. 117.

61.   E. Levin, "Vitamin E vs. Wheat Germ Oil," *American Journal of Digestive Diseases,* Vol. 12. (January 1945), pp. 20-21.

62.   Judith DeCava, p. 54.

63.   Judith DeCava, p. 117.

64.   Judith DeCava, p.161.

65.   Dr. Royal Lee, "The Fallacy of High Potency in Vitamin Dosage."

66.   Brian Scott Peskin, p. 246.

67.   *Medical Tribune:* 36 #22:13, 1995.

68.   Brian Scott Peskin, p. 248.

69.   Dr. Royal Lee, "The Fallacy of High Potency in Vitamin Dosage."

70.   Judith DeCava, M.S., LNC, p. 60.

71.   Dr. Royal Lee, *Vitamin News,* Vol. 6, Feb., 1938, p. 118.

72.   Robert Crayhon, *Robert Crayhon's Nutrition Made Simple* (New York, NY: M. Evans and Co, 1994), p. 80-81.

I have made every effort possible to check the accuracy of material quoted. If there is any question, or a possible mistake in quoting of any material, necessary changes will be made in future printings.

Index

Order Form

Please Print

Name _____

Address _____

City _____ State _____ Zip _____

Phone _____

E-mail _____

METHOD OF PAYMENT

Check _____ Credit Card: Visa_____ Mastercard_____

Card number _____ Exp. date_____

Authorization Signature _____

ITEM	QTY	PRICE
Why Can't I Lose Weight? ($17.95)		
Why Can't I Lose Weight Cookbook ($17.95)		
Why Can't I Stay Motivated? ($14.95)		
Why Am I So Grumpy, Dopey and Sleepy? ($11.95)		
Why Am I So Wacky? ($11.95)		
Why Eat Like Jesus Ate? ($11.95)		
Why Do I Need Whole Food Supplements? ($9.95)		
Why Do I Feel So Lousy? ($9.95)		
Why Do I Really Need Herbs? ($9.95)		
Subtotal		
Shipping & Handling Add 15%		
(Add 8% if resident of OK) Tax		
Total		

Send check or money order to:

Life Design Nutrition

Lorrie Medford, CN

PO Box 54007

Tulsa, OK 74155

918-664-4483

918-664-0300 (fax)

Toll-free 1-877-716-LIFE (5433)

E-mail orders: orders@lifedesignnutrition.com

www.lifedesignnutrition.com